GARY KIRWAN

WINNING A LOSING BATTLE

FROM 41 STONE TO A NEW LIFE

AS HEARD ON **THE RAY D'ARCY SHOW**

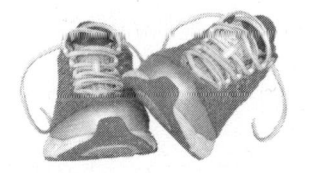

with Nicola Pierce

THE O'BRIEN PRESS
DUBLIN

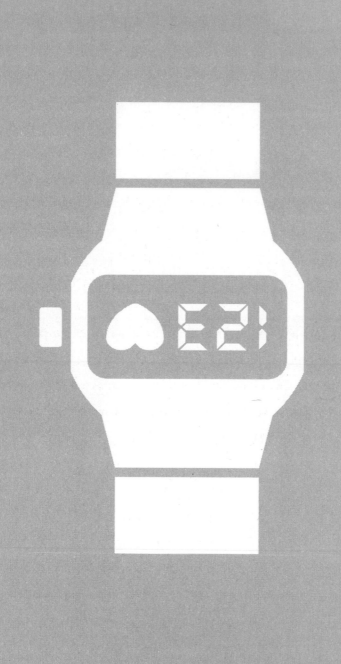

DEDICATION

When I first started writing the diary that eventually became this book, I never knew where it would lead, but I always held the dream of where it might someday end up close to my heart. On my toughest, darkest, hardest days where the diet became extremely hard I could always dream of the one thing I thought I could never have. That dream would always give me a sense of perspective and the determination that the rewards would far outweigh any hardships.

When I started this journey I believed I would never directly father a child, but I hoped that by losing weight it might open other doorways for Shelly and me to have a baby and so I held in my heart the belief that this would one day lead to us seeing this dream becoming a reality.

To our great joy we found out in July that we are pregnant and so the one thing that kept me going when times got tough – our dream – is now reality.

So this book is dedicated to my dream, our unborn child, this has all been for you in the hope that someday I would get to hold you in my arms and love you, to run around with you and to be somebody you can be proud of. I don't think I ever saw it as more than just a dream, but knowing that shortly I will be able to do all of the above makes everything I have done so worthwhile.

So to you I say 'thank you', I already love you so much and you have already done more for me than you will ever realise, you gave me the strength to keep going and you are the greatest reward I could ever receive for my hard work.

Thank you, I can't wait to hold you in my arms.

Love, your dad.

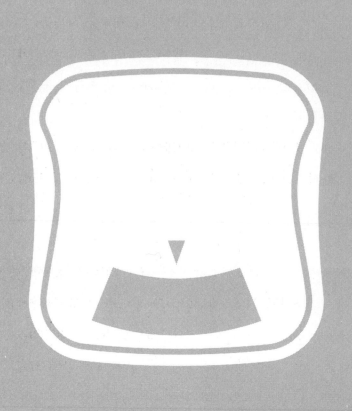

CONTENTS

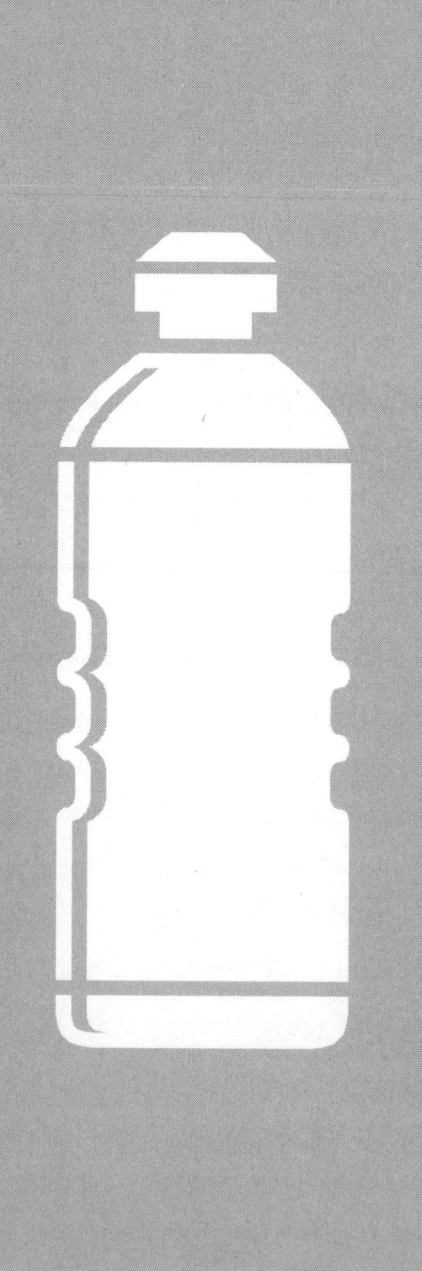

ACKNOWLEDGEMENTS

For over two years I was so lucky to have so much help; I can never thank all those who have helped me enough; your love, support, friendship, encouragement and kindness made this all possible.

Absolutely none of this would ever have taken place if it was not for my beautiful wife and best friend; Shelly, you have been with me every step of the way and have been there for me in good times and bad. You have done so much for me in this. Without you it simply wouldn't have been possible; you are my rock and very soon we will have the rewards for our efforts.

You have always been there in the background doing all the small things that at times go unnoticed and un-thanked, but without which I could not have done so much. You do so much, from boring things like food preparation and getting my training-gear ready, to dealing with the ups and downs of the whole experience. Like a true friend you know when to listen and offer support and you know when to tell me to suck it up, cop on and keep going.

I don't think we ever expected it to be such a big journey and we have had loads of ups and downs, but you kept me going on the tough days and luckily there were more good days than bad. You are always behind me and you have given me so much encouragement. I could not have done this without you. As one journey ends another will soon begin for us and I could not wish for a better friend and wife to share it with.

To my Mam and Dad, Lucia and Peter, who I am lucky to call my friends. Your support has been massively important to me, to see your faces in Dublin was bittersweet as I didn't want you to see me in so much pain, but it kept me going and made me remember how much support and love I have. I know you spent the last few years worrying about me and my health and I am just so happy you will get to see your grandchild grow up and to see Shelly and I as parents. I have learnt from the best and he or she will have such fantastic grandparents. I am both lucky and proud to call you my parents and friends.

If it wasn't for my beautiful niece, Nicole, I don't think I would have had the drive and determination to want a family so much. I don't think this would ever have happened if it were not for you, Nicole. I have enjoyed your company so much over the past few years and on my worst days you were the only thing that made me happy; you're such an amazing little girl. You have brightened up my life so much with your love, kindness, wit and beautiful personality.

To my brothers, sister and their partners, Orla and James, Darren and Ead, Rob and Becky thank you all so much for your love and support over the past two years, it has been greatly appreciated and will never be forgotten. You all got to share in the journey and contributed to it in so many ways and you are all booked in advance for baby-sitting.

To the Carrolls of Loughmore and London, thank you for your support and well wishes over the past few years and thanks for just being there for Shelly and me. To know Shelly has a warm family she can turn to is very comforting; like everybody else you will get to enjoy the next chapter of this story in the years to come.

I would like to thank my aunts, uncles and cousins for all their support over the past two years. I am lucky to have such a great extended family.

To Chris and Carly Delooze: Chris, words can never define how much I appreciate your hard work, friendship and encouragement. You are unlike any other trainer/sportsman/athlete/friend I have ever met and I hope that others are as lucky as I have been to work with you in the future. I really could not have done this without you; when I met you my life took an amazing twist for the better. Thanks also to Carly, Jamie and Corin for allowing Chris to spend so much time helping me, it cannot have been easy at times for you, Carly, but I am glad to say you also shared in some of the high points such as DCM and I thank you so much for allowing Chris time away from his wonderful family to help me. Thanks for everything you have done for me, Chris and Carly.

Tony Browne, you listened to my ups and downs, we had plenty of little chats and it was always great to have your input as you know more than anybody else the demands of such a diet; to have your input was always reassuring, thanks – now get back to work!

To the members of TriFit: thank you all so much. I have always felt part of the gym and considering the high calibre of people/athletes there that is such a great feeling. It has been and always will be a pleasure to be in your company.

I would like to thank the staff of Limerick Charity Boxing, Join Ray for 5k, i3 Swim, Dublin City Marathon, Great Limerick Run, Tri Athy, Fighting Cancer Triathlon, Gaelforce and the Dingle Marathon for your very kind invitations. Knowing I am welcome at an event makes turning up so much easier and through these events I have had some of my best days and experienced a new life. These experiences have given me tremendous strength and your kindness was the first, and probably most important, step in doing these events.

Deccy and Jeff Fitzgerald and family, thank you for your friendship, support and for allowing me to be a part of Limerick Charity Boxing, which has been a very pleasant distraction and gave me my first major goal. It was my first sporting endeavour and it was so enjoyable that it led far beyond a charity boxing event. Thank you also to all the members of Corpus Christi Boxing Club and all those whom I have met through LCB; it has been an absolute pleasure.

Emlyn Maher (physio and friend), I really can't thank you enough for the chats. I am not so sure I can thank you for the pain you inflicted on me, but it kept me going! You have been a massive silent part of this with very little recognition, but it's not really surprising as you are the quiet guy in the background helping everybody else. Thank you so much for all the pain.

Angela Lang, I speak of 'that look' throughout the book, but the look that you gave me was a very different look when we met in Dublin and I am glad to say you have become a friend since DCM and your friendship is very much appreciated.

I would like to thank my classmates and lecturers at Limerick Institute of Technology, I may not be the most sociable person and due to my hectic schedule am always coming and going, but being back in college has been such a pleasant addition to my life.

Thanks to Nichola Forrest (nutritionist) for all your help; you have been the final piece of the puzzle and have helped the whole thing come together. Through your knowledge I am confident that this is now my lifestyle and not just a diet, thank you for all your help and encouragement.

I have had the pleasure of meeting so many others who have helped me throughout the past two years. I really must thank: Denyse O'Brien, Eric Russell, Anna Murphy, Hilary Cleary, Wayne Raphael Reid, Gerry Duffy, Liam & Sophie Mulcahy, Helen and Chris Monoghan, Kay and Frankie Scanlon, Pa Tierney, Thecla Hartmann-Roche, Sharon, Paul, Ger, Miriam, Sinead, Seamus, Rebecca, Margaret, Gary Wilmott and, last but not least, Alicia Ashmore. Thank you all for your support and friendship.

I really could not have done this if it were not for the support I got, so whether it was a kind word at an event or while I was out training, an email, a Facebook message or just a text to Today FM you will probably never realise how that made me feel. Such experiences gave me a whole new outlook on life, which drove me harder to succeed and gave me the encouragement I needed to try new things.

I get a lot of emails from people whose stories are very similar to my own. I always love being able to offer some encouragement through my actions, so much so that nearly all the events I do I do to prove to others that it can be done. I hope by doing some of this it will change people's perception and encourage people just like me to go for it. I just wish I could do more for those who have emailed me. I am always humbled by your stories and kind words.

To Michael O'Brien and his team at The O'Brien Press, thank you for giving me this opportunity to tell my story in detail; while it is still very surreal it has been a very pleasant and therapeutic experience for me.

The Motivation Weight Management Clinic who for the first twelve months helped me with my diet.

Thanks Nicola Pierce (co-writer) for helping me with this, it has been a pleasure to work with you – I hope it hasn't been too stressful!

Last, but by no means least, thanks to the people who made it all happen (I know Ray will say, 'But sure we didn't do anything!'), but that is simply not true. For many years I have listened to the *Ray D'Arcy Show* and, like a lot of people, Ray and his team became a part of my life – so much so that I turned to you for help. Walking into studio on 17 January was terrifying, but at least I felt I had met you before so I felt a little bit comfortable. From day one Ray and his team showed me compassion, support and an overwhelming amount of kindness. So much so that I felt comfortable talking about what lay in the darkest parts of my heart. Through your interviews I have grown and shrunk in so many ways. I can never thank Ray, Jenny, Mairead, Will, Pam, Roisín and Siobhan, who have all been part of this for over two years, enough. I know you will all say you did nothing, but you gave me kindness and the opportunity to talk openly, which has, in many ways, become my therapy. I truly believe I could not have done this without you and from the bottom of my heart I thank you all for everything. I had a lot of contact with Jenny and Siobhan in particular and I would like to say 'thank you so much' to you both, you really went above and beyond and have always been there for me, which was such a massive safety net as I always had your support. Thank you both so much. A special thanks to the warmth I have been shown by the staff of Today FM: the smiles, kind words and even the odd round of applause was always so much appreciated when I was leaving studio. Thank you for adding to the experience with your kindness.

As you can see, I should really be writing a book about all the great people I have had the pleasure of meeting (maybe it could be the sequel!) and who have helped me over the past two years. I have been so lucky to have had so much support. It has been incredible to go from where I was in life to having so many people rooting for me.

To all of you who have shared this journey with me, thank you all so much, no matter how small a part you played it was always very much appreciated and I hope to able to repay your kindness in the years to come.

FOREWORD
BY RAY D'ARCY

Back in January 2011 we got a run of the mill email into 'Fix it Friday' asking could we locate a weighing scales for a listener's husband. He was too heavy to use a domestic scales and desperately wanted to know his weight. All he knew was that he was over 30 stone. That woman was Shelly and the man was Gary Kirwan. Gary came in to us and asked to do a live weigh-in on the industrial scales we had located from a company in Naas. Gary was a big man. He was out of breath when he arrived to studio after little or no exertion and throughout our initial chat his breathing was laboured. From the off two things were obvious to me: he was determined and he was eloquent.

Gary immediately struck a chord with our listeners. His story of being grossly overweight and everything that goes with it was a sad story. He wasn't well physically or mentally either. The latter was on the up. When the moment came for Gary to step up on the scales, neither of us knew that this was to become a regular feature of the radio show for the next eighteen months and more. Around 35 stone was Gary's guesstimate of his weight. He was wrong. Six stone wrong. Gary weighed in at 41 stone.

After the collective shock abated we heard how Gary aimed to reduce that to around 16 stone – that's a weight loss of 25 stone. That's more than two of me. Gary hasn't achieved his goal yet, but he has achieved, I believe, much more. 'Inspirational' is an overused word in a world where we have to remind ourselves of the word's true meaning. Gary Kirwan is inspirational. Gary finishing the Dublin Marathon in darkness, after walking for 10 hours and 46 minutes, was a truly Herculean achievement. Gary Kirwan is impressive. He talks the talk and walks the walk. He was always very honest and frank about the ups and downs of his weight loss.

Since day one, Gary has kept a 'warts and all' diary of his life, which now provides the basis of this book. I know you will be impressed by Gary's determination, discipline and downright doggedness in his attempt to achieve his weight-loss goal.

RAY D'ARCY

I DON'T BLAME ANYBODY ELSE FOR MY WEIGHT, I AM RESPONSIBLE FOR MY WEIGHT. NOBODY ELSE, ME.

MY DECISIONS OVER THE YEARS WERE POOR, OFTEN THEY WERE NOT EVEN CONSIDERED AND VERY STUPID; I MADE FOOLISH DECISIONS, BUT ULTIMATELY THEY WERE MY DECISIONS.

I HAVE LOST A HUGE PART OF MY LIFE, GONE THROUGH THINGS THAT I WISH I HAD NOT; I HAVE HAD TO LIVE IN SHAME OF THE PERSON I HAD BECOME.

THIS IS MY STORY OF HOW I GOT TO 41 STONE 3 POUNDS AND HOW I AM GETTING MYSELF OUT OF IT. IT IS NOT A DIET BOOK, IT IS JUST MY STORY.

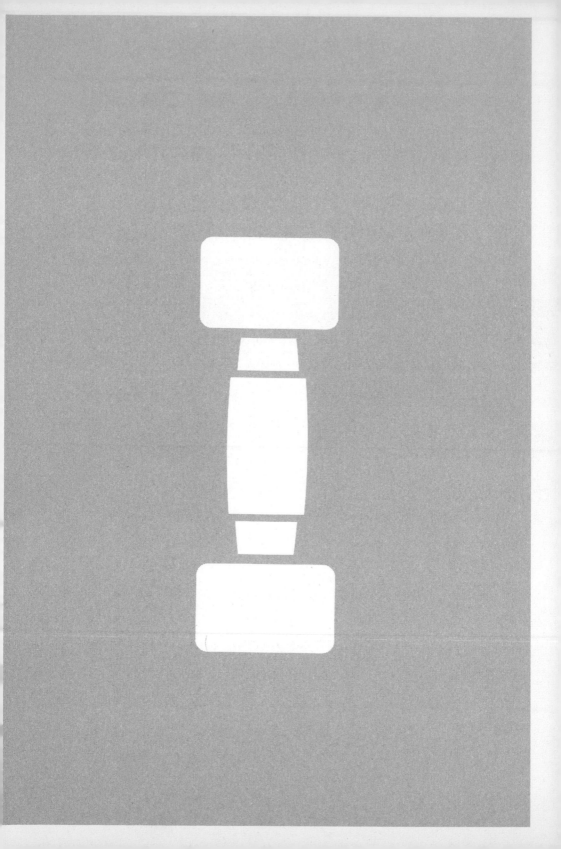

'IF I DO NOT GIVE UP I CANNOT FAIL'

This quote means an awful lot to me. I found it in relation to a piece I've watched on YouTube – many, many times. In fact, I would well believe that I am responsible for at least a thousand viewings of the clip. It's from the 1992 Olympics, which were held in Barcelona, and features the British runner Derek Redmond. He held the British record for the 400 metre sprint and won gold medals at the World Championships, European Championships as well as the Commonwealth games. So, you can imagine that he was a popular favourite for a medal at the 1992 games.

I can only guess the hours, days, weeks and months of training that went into preparing him for standing at that start line in Barcelona. The crowd was huge, about 65,000 watching the runners stretch their legs and then line up, their faces a study in tense concentration. It is all about winning, or, at the very least, doing the very best you can do, no matter what.

At last, the gun is fired and the runners take off, chasing themselves and their dream of an Olympic medal. Redmond is looking strong and powerful, until, that is, about 150 metres into the race when something goes wrong. Suddenly he is clutching his leg in agony and coming to a shocking standstill as his competitors overtake and leave him behind forevermore, as far as that race is concerned. He falls to the ground, his body utterly gripped by the pain caused by a torn hamstring. And you might think, well, that's it then. God love him!

But you would be wrong.

Somehow, he finds the brutal strength to stand up … and then, unbelievably, he starts limping forward, his injury forcing him to sort of hop along a track he'd only experienced as a champion sprinter. His face expresses more than a thousand words could – sheer pain, sadness and raw emotion. You can sense the bewilderment of the crowd and the race officials. One guy approaches him, no doubt to help the stricken runner off to the side, but Redmond keeps going. I am sure that everyone is wondering what the hell is going on.

And Redmond just keeps going.

For a couple of breathtaking minutes he is alone in the world, with his pain and his incessant need to keep moving forward. However, this 'aloneness' is just temporary. A grey-haired man, in a white tee-shirt, his face full of concern, rushes out to his side. It's Redmond's father, who was seated in the crowd and has had to break through tight security in order to get to his son.

His father says what everyone else is probably thinking, 'You don't have to do this!' Redmond's answer is immediate and solid, 'Yes … I do.' Without wasting another second in debating this, his father takes him by the arm and tells him, 'Well, then we will finish it together'. The two men keep going, at a snail's pace and, by this stage, the crowd realise what they are looking at … courage and spirit, an Olympic spirit that has nothing to do with winning.

Just before the finish line, Mr Redmond does the right and honourable thing; he releases his son so that he can cross over the line, alone once more. Those sixty-five thousand are now on their feet, roaring their support and admiration. Derek Redmond may not have won a medal that year, but I think you'll agree that medals, in this case, are hardly the point.

So, that is what I watched, night after night, when things got really tough. I suppose not many people have stood on a weighing scale and had to read that they were 41 stone. At the beginning of my journey, my own personal race, I had an awful lot to do, in terms of losing stones of weight and the psychological weight that my massiveness involved. There was a time when I wouldn't leave the house, for fear of people staring at me, pointing at me, calling me names. Things, I'm glad to say, are a lot different now. But it has not been easy.

At the end of this video is the epic tagline that has become my mantra: 'If I do not give up I cannot fail'. I quite simply decided if I don't give up I won't fail. What I most admired about Derek Redmond is not the medals he won, but that he had the heart of a lion.

I'm not an Olympic athlete. When I turn up to take part in sporting events I have a fair idea that I may end up coming in last, or in the bottom few, but it doesn't bother me. And while I may not win, nobody, including myself, can doubt my trying. As far as I see it, I'm already beating the thousands of others who won't even take their place at the start line.

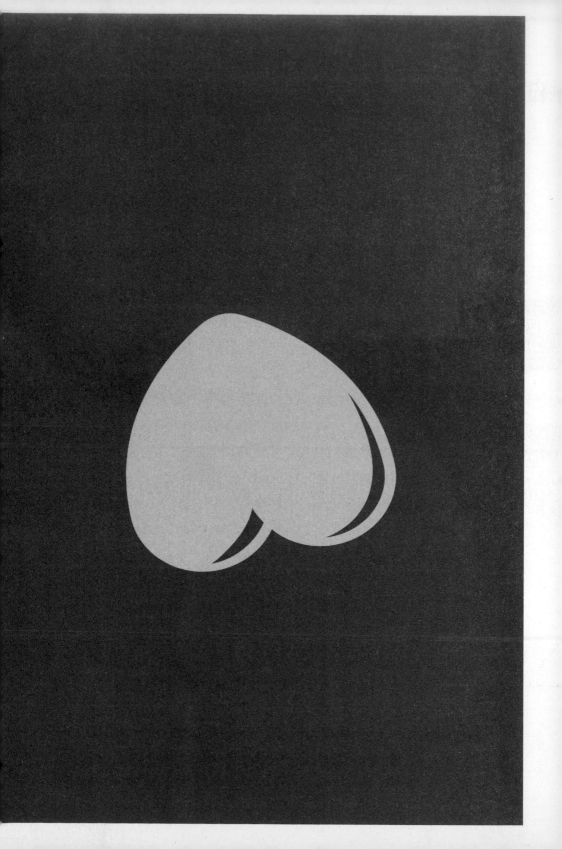

PART

ONE

EARLY YEARS

There isn't a time that I can remember *not* being big. They say that everything begins at home, so let's start there. I am the second oldest in a family of four, with one older sister, Orla, and two younger brothers, Darren and Rob, who were all slim to skinny. The youngest did go through a patch of puppy fat, which he rapidly lost on discovering the opposite sex. My dad, a mechanic, and a dead ringer for *Emmerdale's* Eric Pollard, is small and of normal build, while my mother, a born teacher and organiser, was always skinny.

For the first fourteen years of my life we lived in a small cul-de-sac, in Richmond Park, Corbally. At that time we were surrounded by green fields and it was a great place to be. There were loads of kids, aged six to sixteen, so there was always something going on, with loads to do. Plenty of football matches were played on our street or else we were up to mischief in the fields. When the building started, with new houses and estates going up, around us, these building sites became a haven for games of hide and seek.

My earliest memory is of the classroom that Mam set up in our house, in Limerick. There she minded us and other kids from the area. That classroom had everything you would expect to see. I loved anything to do with arts and crafts and created wonderful pieces of sculpture from the plasticine, or '*mála*', that my mother made especially for us.

Later on she set up a 'Play Scheme', with her friend, Vera, in St Mary's girls' school. It was a summer camp before there were summer camps, run by local parents for the local kids. I don't remember much about it, other than I loved it. Though I do remember taking part in a fancy dress competition, in 1985, the year that Barry McGuigan won the world title. I went as the Clones Cyclone, even going as far as blacking up my eye with soot from the chimney. My interest in boxing must have begun back then.

Money was always tight although we never wanted for anything. Therefore, a visit to Burgerland, Limerick's version of McDonalds, was a rarity saved up for birthdays or equally special occasions. We didn't get takeaways and our only real treat was the glass of fizzy drink and chocolate bar that we had on Saturday nights, in front of the television. I pretty much ate the same as my sister and brothers, our school lunches consisted of a sandwich, Penguin bar and a packet of crisps. However, I will say this; I ate faster than anyone else in the house. My poor mother was always on at me to slow down at meal times, but I never did.

It annoys me when people talk about families that enable children to become obese. My mother did not over-feed me and, yet, it turned out that I got fat while the brother next to me was always as skinny as a rake.

There was an incident that, thankfully, I have no memory of, as I was only five years old. Vera, my mother's friend, had a teenaged daughter called Niamh who, from time to time, would take us kids swimming. The story goes that one day, on our return, she was very upset and had to be cajoled into explaining that some other children in the pool had been laughing and making crude jokes about me. As I say, I was just a five-year-old having fun and, therefore, was completely oblivious to their sneering.

I suppose my earliest memory about realising that my weight was an issue came two years later. It was 1987 and I was making my First Holy Communion. Mam took me out to buy my suit, bringing me to Noel's Menswear, in town, where just about everyone I knew went to buy their communion outfits. Unfortunately they didn't have a suit in my size so we were forced to traipse around a few other shops that catered for communion, confirmations and even men's shops, before my mother gave up. Naturally I had little or no interest in wearing a suit; my favourite outfit, at that time, was my trusty tracksuit. In the end Mam had to go to a tailor and have a suit specially made for me, in green khaki. I'm only appreciating now, as I write this, that it must have cost a fortune. However, none of this unexpected fuss prevented me from enjoying my special day. There was a tradition in our family that when any of us made our communion or confirmation we went to our neighbours, the Scanlon's, for lunch. Then, when the Scanlon kids had their day, they came to our house for lunch. We all got on well together, kids and adults, and it was always great fun. A grand total of fourteen of these lunches took place, over the years, between their family and ours, all of which were amazing days out with some great memories.

But, of course, more importantly I also made a small fortune, touring the relatives, in my green custom-made suit, enough to be allowed, at any rate, to blow some of it at my favourite toy shop.

Do kids still go mad about tennis the way we did back then? Once we had our fill of Wimbledon, watching the likes of John McEnroe and Martina Navratilova, all the local kids would fling themselves into the Kit Kat tennis summer camp. Like tennis, the camp would only last two weeks. I was never very good at the game but I still enjoyed myself as much as anyone else.

My primary school was Scoil Íde, and the years I spent there were pleasant enough. I liked my teachers even if I was bored by school work itself. Perhaps thanks to my mother's play school my one and only favourite subject was art and crafts. At home I could spend hours building elaborate designs with my Lego and Meccano set. Fortunately I always had a great imagination, which I relied on to escape from the boredom of maths, Irish and pretty much everything else in school. People like children to read so that it will stimulate their imagination, but I never had much interest in books myself, even though our house was always full of them because my parents were, and still are, great readers.

When my Dad and his brother, Tommy, were young, they would come home via the local bookshop every Friday, armed with their reading for the weekend. On a few occasions the two men even rang in sick on Monday so that they could finish the book they were reading. Most nights my mother retired to bed with a book in her hands. Maybe it is a little strange that I did not inherit a love for this particular past-time, but there it is, I never had the least bit of interest in reading. I much preferred to look at pictures in the books and make up my own stories about them.

My spelling was always very poor. I could get the first and last letter of a word but the middle bit would be jumbled up, which concerned my mother. When I was about eight years old, she had me checked out and it was discovered I was slightly dyslexic. However, I did not suffer over it. I attended special classes, within the school day, for children with learning difficulties. I loved this class. The teacher was a Mary Kennedy who really understood how to relate to kids who were not into learning that much. It was like she taught us stuff without us even realising it.

Of course I was the big kid all through primary school but it was never an issue. Young kids don't realise that they might have the power to upset a classmate, and get a kick out of doing it – that comes later. The only thing I truly hated about school back then was the annual sports day. Every year I came last in front of an audience made up of the entire school, including staff, which was embarrassing. As you might imagine, I could not wait for that particular day to finish. Though there was this one time, when I was in fifth or sixth class, and I was standing at the start line for the sprint; naturally I did not fancy my chances one little bit. The teacher blew the whistle and I took off, relatively speaking. Within a matter of seconds I was bewildered by the fact that I could not see any of my fellow sprinters in front of me. I was so used to spending races puffing along while having the time to study the backs of the other competitors. It turned out that the boys were behind me, walking slowly to allow me, I think, a shot at winning something for a change. Unfortunately the teacher spoilt the fun by calling us all back to re-start the race and things went back to normal: I was about twenty metres into the race while the rest were over the finish line and catching their breath.

But then my weight did become an issue, and one that could no longer be ignored by my worried parents. In April 1991 I had to have an operation to remove a testicle from my stomach. I was ten years old. It is a common enough occurrence, or so I'm told, and has nothing to do with weight. The matter has to be rectified before puberty hits or it can affect one's fertility later on. However, what made my experience distinctive was hearing the surgeon a few weeks later, at my check-up, telling Mam that he had never had to cut through so much fat on a child. He advised her to have something done about it and made a few suggestions. All I cared about was the two toy wrestlers I got for being a good patient.

My mother had always been fairly strict about what I ate, but I think this worried her and it resulted in her bringing me to see a dietician in Limerick Regional Hospital. Now, at this point I would like to interject and again say that I was not eating loads and loads of crap with my parents' blessing. Yes, I sneaked things from presses in between meals, but there would not have been too exciting a range of 'bad' food to help myself to. My mother did her best to make sure I snacked on fruit and healthy stuff like yoghurts. The only day of the week I had chips was on a Thursday when we had our chicken and chips dinner. Darren, my skinny brother, ate really slowly and maybe that helped him to feel full for longer than I did. If I felt bored or lonely, at this age, I did not go and stuff my face. I enjoyed my meals, but I did race through them as if I could win a medal to make up for the poor showing I gave at the school's sports' days. My one failing was fizzy drinks. If I had money to spend it usually went on Coke or Fanta, stuff like that.

Looking back now I can see how the diet programme at the hospital could not have helped me at all. I suppose not a lot was known back then about child obesity, or whatever you like to call it. The dietician, a lady, was nice but she never asked me about myself or my personal eating habits. Instead we came away with a ton of booklets, about diet and so forth, that were aimed at the masses. There was no interest in particular cases, like that of a ten-year-old boy who somehow was the heaviest in his slim family. She never thought to ask me if I was unhappy, or why I was always hungry. Meanwhile, the diet, in my opinion, was just plain wrong, in that it advocated lots of carbohydrates. So I ate lots of potato, bread, pasta and rice, thinking it was going to help me lose weight. I had to cut out sugar, but sure there was little or no weight loss thanks to the amount of carbs I was eating every day.

Maybe with a bit more knowledge and curiosity, the dietician might have discovered something that I only found out in the last eighteen months – grains do not suit my body. But that is probably unfair of me. She was following the rules set out in those brochures and would not have considered, like my mother and me, to question them.

I was to spend the next five years trying to lose weight on this diet, with frequent visits to the dietician. Since I never actually lost much weight it was frustrating for all involved – as well as being demoralising for me, in fact I put up weight gradually over this period.

CHAPTER TWO

SCHOOL DAYS

I started secondary school in 1992, in CBS Sexton Street, Limerick. I was in the class group that did the more hands-on subjects like woodwork, art and technical drawing. After my Inter Cert I had the option to go into a more academic stream, but I was adamant I wanted to do these subjects. The class had around forty boys or young men in First Year; by the Leaving Cert only fifteen of us remained. It was a bit of an eye-opener as there were some real characters in the class! On starting in Sexton Street, once again I was the fat kid but, this time, there were a few others too, it was a big school. The furniture was against me from the very beginning. Except for Second Year we had the old-style wooden desks, where the bench and desk are connected, and, ordinarily, there is room for two. I remember feeling sorry for Keith Prendergast, he shared my desk with me in First Year and it must have been a bit of a squeeze for him, but, to be fair to him, he never said anything.

First and Second Year went by without too much trouble. I was slagged over my size but it was just boys being boys, in that everyone, at one stage, got a ribbing over something. In First Year I took up hurling with a passion that was unequalled by the other, far superior players. In fact, I would go so far as to say that I was quite probably the worst hurler that every represented the school, but I genuinely loved the game – not least because matches meant half days from the classroom.

The ninety-minute PE (Physical Education) class was a very long one for me. As far as I remember, we seemed to do the 'bleep test' – a fitness test where we had to run between two points at ever decreasing time intervals – very frequently in First Year. I was always the first to be knocked out in anything that involved speed, so I usually spent the best part of that hour sitting on the bench with Allan Franklin, a skinny kid who hated PE as much as I did, but I think it was for very different reasons, he just didn't like it and I was crap at it. We would watch the others, in silence, feeling that time was crawling to a standstill.

I was still an avid day-dreamer, mentally removing myself from boring classes and running entire films in my head based on whatever cartoons I was watching at the time. It was all too easy for me to completely switch off and spend forty minutes as a super hero or sports star, while one teacher or another droned on, and on, about algebra or Irish grammar. Naturally, in these dreams, since I was both the director and producer I played the starring role, and was always super fit, strong and very, very fast. I certainly was not the chubby kid squeezed into a desk that barely contained me and poor Keith.

And the thing about it is that I did not worry about being chubby, fat, or how I looked, since I had always been that way as far as I could remember. It was part of who I was. It was me. I am sure that it is fair to say that when I looked in the mirror, there were days when I might have hated the flabby person staring back at me, but then there were the days that I merely needed to check my reflection, to see if my hair was okay or my face was clean, before I left the house, and I would not have noticed my bigness, any more than I might have noticed my eyebrows. Other kids might fret about their acne or their height, or – especially boys – if feel they are too small, or look much younger than their friends, but they forget about it too, and get on with their day. We are allowed to forget about ourselves, up to a point, the point being when something happens outside of us, when we are suddenly shocked into viewing ourselves through another person's eyes. The shock depends, I suppose, on who that person is.

My point was reached in Third Year. I was fifteen years old.

By this stage I was wearing heavy jumpers all the time, to hide my man-boobs. Out of sight, out of mind, and jumpers, I quickly discovered, formed the perfect barrier between me, the general public and my sagging chest, which was extremely embarrassing. They had always been there, but once I hit puberty they just grew and grew and I was extremely self-conscious about them. No matter how hot it got, or what month it was, nothing could make me take off my jumper. The school uniform involved a jumper, bearing the school's crest. Now, this should have been glad tidings for me except for the fact that school jumpers might well be the most unforgiving of all jumpers in the jumper-world. Anyone who ever had to wear one, and was not built like a bean-pole, will know exactly what I mean. I know they are made from wool, so why is it that they cling to a body like a leotard, or a wet swim suit?

Brother Power was the principal and he was a typical one in that we were mostly terrified of him, for good reason, but he also had a decent side. It was my mother who approached him, she wrote to him about my problem regarding the school jumper. The brother carried a bit of weight himself, and I think this is why he immediately allowed me to wear a substitute navy jumper of my own, the only solution available to me. When I think about it now I really appreciate his kindness, as it could well have gone the other way, where I might have been forced to do without and go about in the white flimsy school shirt, which would have left nothing to the imagination. The problem was solved and I took to wearing a navy fleece that stretched over me nicely, with my principal's blessing. It allowed me to hide my embarrassment; for a young man of around fourteen it was a huge embarrassment to have man-boobs bigger than most girls of the same age.

One afternoon my class was waiting for our usual teacher to arrive, I can't remember which one, when the door opened and a man we did not know strode purposefully to the desk, shouting at us to be quiet. Maybe our teacher was sick, I don't know, but this guy was ready for trouble. Our class did have a lot of messers in it, and he was taking no hostages. It's strange, but I remember this as if it had just happened ten minutes ago; you know how there is always one scene from your childhood that stays with you forever and ever? Well, this is mine. He was very tanned, wore grey slacks, white shirt and glasses, had a real 'prim and proper' look about him – and he was as skinny as a rake.

He fired insults left, right and centre, obviously needing to establish from the very beginning that he was the boss and we were just a bunch of no-good hoodlums: 'You sit down!', 'Shut up you!', 'You, there, take off that jumper!' That last one was flung at me, where I was sitting, at the back of the room. I jumped, 'Sir?' All eyes turned to me as he repeated himself, in a voice dripping with contempt, 'I said, take off that jumper. It's not school uniform'. I am sure I must have been blushing furiously as I tried to explain that I was allowed to wear what I was wearing, 'Brother Power says it's all right'. As far as I was concerned, and any other of my fellow pupils, they were the magic words, just like the words 'Open Sesame' opened up the cave in the story of 'Ali Baba and the Forty Thieves' : *Brother Power says it's all right.* End of story. Only it wasn't. I don't think I can quite describe the horror I experienced on hearing him reply, 'You are in my classroom. Here, we play by my rules!' It was utterly bewildering. This was not *his* classroom; none of us had ever seen him before and even if it was his classroom – which it wasn't – Brother Power was the one in charge of all of us, not him. Panic set in, along with a bitter surge of helplessness. He was the teacher while I was just an unruly pupil who had absolutely no chance of evading his direct order. It was horrible, that slow dawning that, at this point, I had no option but to remove my fleece, my barrier, my safety net. I hated myself for giving in but, really, what else could I do? I was taught at home to be well-behaved and so was in no way prepared to stand my ground against a teacher.

He sat down at the desk and reached for his newspaper while I slowly took the bottom of my fleece in my two hands and miserably began to lift it towards my head. I cannot remember if I was aware that the rest of the class were watching me do this – however, it soon became abundantly clear that they were watching when, somehow, I managed to pull my shirt up, along with the fleece, thereby exposing my belly, by far the biggest in the room, for all to see. Everyone started to laugh at me, including the teacher. The sound of his chuckle and the laughter of the class haunted me for weeks, months after. He silently gave the class permission and his approval to see my size as a source of entertainment. What could I do but continue to remove my fleece, as the boys around me laughed and laughed. He said something, I don't know what, but whoever heard it bellowed even louder. When I looked up at him, all I could see was the top of his head, behind the newspaper, shaking with laughter … at me.

This might not sound like much, but I am crying as I write this down. That was the worst day of my childhood and probably my life. Everything changed, from this point onwards. Up to then I never really considered my body as something to be considered by anyone else. What that man did was open my eyes, and everyone else's, to the fact that my bigness was apart from me. Those boys had known me for years and were, no doubt, accustomed to me, not giving my belly a second thought. I was Gary Kirwan, a person first and foremost, and it was all part of the package. In those few seconds that teacher taught them to look at me differently, almost separating the boy they knew from the big body. Even now I hate myself for not, at the very least, having the guts to walk out of that room – however, I know I'm being unfair to myself. I was only fifteen years old and did not make a habit of causing scenes in school, as I had been raised not to. From that day forward I became both an emotional eater and a constant target for more than just a bit of slagging.

A lot of readers might be wondering what I might have been eating at the time and I understand that. I don't like focusing too much on food itself. People put on weight without thinking about it and I'm sure plenty would agree with me when I say that it is the easiest thing in the world to do. So I don't have any scandalous confessions to make regarding eating entire cakes or packs of biscuits. For the most part this sort of stuff wasn't to be found in my mother's presses. All I did was get used to eating in between meals. When I came home from school I accidentally got used to eating before my dinner. What started out as one sandwich became two sandwiches, or I would start pouring myself out big bowls of breakfast cereal ... a couple of hours later I would have my dinner. It is as easy as that.

Around the time I was in First Year, Weightwatchers came to Limerick and my mother decided I should join. I think we had both given up on the dietician and the brochures, from the hospital, and were ready to try something new. The Weightwatchers meetings took place in the Glentworth Hotel and Mam came with me for moral support for the first few weeks, for which I was very grateful. I hardly knew what to expect. When we arrived at the hotel it was all women, or else I just cannot remember seeing any men around. I was the youngest by far, and I also have a strong memory of the fact that nobody looked as heavy as I did; in fact I can't remember anybody bar myself being obviously overweight.

In fact their diet wasn't too different from the dietician's. We were allowed three meals a day and two snacks. I went once a week; Mam accompanied me the first few times until I was ready to go by myself. To be honest it did not make much of an impact on me. Looking back, I would probably make the same point that I made about the dietician, the diet was not specific enough for me, a thirteen-year-old schoolboy.

I followed the plans rigidly, which resulted in Mam having to make me a different dinner from everyone else, and, yet, I don't remember losing much, if any weight.

Things got pretty bad about two months into Fifth Year. The slagging, the name calling turned into out and out bullying. I began to feel that every day was the same; I was the butt of all jokes in the classroom. I did my best to ignore it, but if you have to listen to stuff every day, five days a week, sooner or later you are bound to crack. I was never a tough guy, I wouldn't have known where to start, so I think I must have surprised myself more than anyone, when one afternoon I had taken just about enough of the constant abuse. We were in class, I can't remember which subject, when one of my usual tormenters laughed out loud at some joke cracked by one of his mates, about me, and I just saw red. I would love to be able to describe a much better fight than the one I gave him, but the truth of it is that I would have stumbled over to him and thrown a couple of messy punches – I was a very inexperienced fighter – that he easily protected himself from. His mate separated us and the teacher threw us both out of the room. It wasn't a glorious moment, I'll grant you, but it was an important one for me, since it was the very first time that I had stood up for myself and I silently vowed it wouldn't be the last.

Once the bullying started I distanced myself from the others, choosing to spend most of my free time alone. I began to hate the school. At home I put on a brave face. Nobody knew I was being bullied, nobody knew exactly how miserable I was. After that first fight there were a few more. It was mostly the job of two boys, in particular, to constantly pick on me and call me names. There was a popular computer game that featured a character called 'Big Boy Barry' and that became my new name – when I wasn't being called after some massive wrestler. Then there were the jokes, the innuendoes, and I'm glad I cannot remember any of them. I just remember feeling exhausted with the non-stop attention. Anytime I let down my guard they were at me, nibbling away at what was left of my confidence. I felt worthless, that is the simplest way I can put it … utterly worthless. When their audience laughed, it served as a horrible reminder of that day when the entire class had laughed along with that teacher. It was like an open wound that never had a chance to heal.

I think it is important to say that not everybody in my class set out to make my life hell, maybe just one or two people in particular and one or two more joined in from time to time, but by this stage I was around twenty stone, had acne and man boobs and they managed to find plenty of entertainment in that, while it was just these few individuals that made the bulk of the jokes most people laughed at them – or at least it felt that way to me.

A few weeks after that first fight, I walked out of the school, in the middle of the day, walked home, let myself into the house and told my parents that I wanted to leave school immediately. There had been another explosion of laughter at my expense and I thought to myself, *That's it, no more.* Naturally they asked me why, and, for some reason, I could not tell them the truth about what was going on, what I was dealing with on a daily basis. Instead I just said that I hated school – which, I realise, is not much of a reason for anything. I hadn't the heart to tell them how bad things had gotten. It was some sort of primal instinct to want to keep them from knowing how much pain I was in.

I wouldn't have upset or worried either of them for the world.

Well, education was important to them so there was no way that they could agree to me leaving school in fifth year. In those days you were nothing without the Leaving Certificate, and I knew that as well as anyone else. I don't think I really believed that they would have let me leave; I probably just needed to do something, that day, to get away from the torment. Sometimes I wish now that I had told them the truth. They made me go back to school but, after a while, it all got on top of me again, so I did what was necessary. Each morning, I'd put on my uniform, have my breakfast, pick up my school-bag and say goodbye to Mam and head to school. When the slagging started, as it invariably did, I'd simply leave, 'mitch', and then make my way to the canal, which was nearby. There I'd spend the day dreaming and pottering around until it was time to go home again. I must have done that for the next year and a half. The strange thing is I was never missed, nobody at school ever wondered where I was.

However it wasn't all bad. I did take up rugby, around this time. I was a prop – well, let's face it; I was never going to be a scrum half. I played on the under-16 and under-18 team for Young Munsters, and, for once, my size appeared to be a good thing that I could benefit from. My parents were delighted; they were always encouraging me to get involved in sports. I was probably the most dedicated member of the team. Whatever the weather, it didn't matter; I never missed one training session. I went twice a week and it was up to Mam or Dad to drive me there and back, since the rugby grounds were on the other side of town.

I was never very good at it. I mean, I loved it and enjoyed the training but as the team got better and better I found myself losing my place for the matches to other superior players who hardly turned up for training. Whatever about my hefty size being a good thing for a prop, I was much too slow, much too unfit to be of any real use. Chappie, the coach, was always very good to me and did his best to encourage me; he took a bit of an interest in me and was always trying to encourage me to lose the weight. Again the uniform presented a problem for me. I had to convince my parents to buy me an expensive jersey, since the ones on offer, for the team, were much too small. I was still very paranoid about my man-boobs; even the expensive jersey was useless in camouflaging them. Mam bought me a rubber belt that was supposed to be worn about the stomach and helped to make you sweat. I figured it would help me get rid of the boobs and possibly make them appear smaller in the meantime.

I'll never forget my last day of playing rugby for the team. We had made it to the semi-final of the under-18s cup, to play Shannon RFC at the Tom Clifford Park. Needless to say it was an important match for us, a very big deal indeed. It was a close, tense match and I spent most of it on the bench until about ten minutes from the end when Chappie kindly gave me a chance to play (one of the props got injured and I was put on). The pace was fast, with plenty of sprinting and chasing, and I just could not keep up with the others. My lack was severely highlighted when, a few minutes before the final whistle, there was a ruck near the Shannon line and we had the chance to win the match if we could score a try. I was coming towards the ruck I should have stayed away, but to be honest I was out on my feet and I wasn't thinking. The scrum half passed the ball out when I was running in and the ball came off my leg – I had knocked it on and gave away a penalty. We lost possession and the match. As you might imagine I felt bloody awful and hung my head in shame. I don't think I ever felt so lonely in my life as when the referee sounded the end, to resounding applause from the Shannon team and supporters. I dreaded heading back into the changing rooms and couldn't look at my team-mates. It was only to be expected that a few guys on the team turned on me, to vent their frustration, making some nasty comments about my lack of skill and my man-boobs. That was the last match of the season and my last day playing for Young Munsters, I didn't totally give up and instead joined St Mary's rugby club and while my skill didn't improve it was a much more pleasant experience.

Over the summer between Fifth and Sixth Year I piled on the weight; I just ate and ate. At times it was the only thing that made me happy. I was so miserable, so I was also aggressive and short-tempered, which caused problems at home as I argued with my brothers and sisters. Mam and Dad did everything possible to try and get me to eat better, but I hid what was going on very well. I had always worked; from as young as fifteen I always had jobs, from a paper round to working in a factory and as Christmas staff in Dunnes, which is why I had money to buy food that I wouldn't have got at home.

Sixth Year: I was seventeen years old and twenty-three stone. When I last weighed less than my age, I could not remember. A couple of months before the Leaving Certificate I filled out my CAO forms. I applied for a course at the Limerick Institute of Technology (LIT), and went along to the Open Day. Once again I was not allowed to forget myself. The night before the Open Day, there had been a film on TV in which one of the characters was called 'Lard Ass'. I was standing with a group of would-be students in the main hall of the college; we were being given a tour around the place. The hall was quite crowded, and, though I was shy, it felt good to be part of the buzzing atmosphere. It was so different from school, and a chance for a new beginning after all those months spent by the canal. Suddenly I became aware of a sort of chant being directed at me. A group of country lads had obviously seen the film and were now gleefully shouting 'Lard Ass' at me, over and over again. Of course everyone in the hall turned to see what the commotion was and who the source of it was. People stared, some giggled. I know I pretended to laugh along, to be a good sport. Inside, however, I was feeling crushed once more.

That April, just after the incident in LIT and a couple of months before my exams, I had told my mother that I wanted to lose weight, and this time I was serious. Starting college in September was my motivation. I'd had enough of the sneering and having to fake laughter at myself in order to fit in. It was time to take control of my life, of my body. After the years with the dietician and Weightwatchers we decided to try an allergy test. It did not make sense that I never lost weight despite sticking rigidly to whatever diet sheet was given to me. There had to be a reason for this. Neither Mam nor I knew much about nutrition but when we heard about this new thing, an allergy test to see if there were problem foods for a particular individual, it seemed like the perfect step to take. As a result of the test I cut out chocolate, corn, pork, beef and foods that contained Monosodium glutamate (MSG), a commonly-used additive which enhances the flavour of savoury products, from tomato pastes to soups, and so on. Funnily enough, the test did not make mention of any problems with bread and grains, nor did it mention anything about fizzy drinks

I cut out everything as per the allergy test and over a few weeks the weight fell off, but then I started to want to lose weight even faster and would just eat less, which ultimately turned into a starvation diet of sorts. I ate as little as I could; I hated what my life had become and I wanted to start my college life as a new person. I would no longer indulge my appetite or feel the least bit sorry for myself, which, in the past, had only led to me to eating large bowls of breakfast cereal and one or even two sandwiches, in between my dinner and lunch. No, sir. I cut all that out, went cold turkey and proved to be a ruthless hard task-master on myself. When I felt pain from hunger I considered this to be a very good thing that propelled me to keep going. I ate very little, if at all, and I also turned to exercise, in the form of cycling. I headed out early in the mornings, when the roads were at their quietest, and sometimes a second time, in the afternoons. I am not a person who believes in doing things by half. Hell-bent on a new me, I courted physical pain, light-headedness and mostly felt quite ill from a severe lack of sustenance. In no way did it occur to me that what I was doing was bad for my health, even dangerous. All I thought about was losing weight, as fast as I could. When I felt really sick I would eat skittles to keep me going. I had heard that rugby players take skittles before a match for a sugar-rush so I took to eating a handful when I felt really tired or dizzy.

Well, I lost weight all right, my first big loss. By the time I started in Limerick School of Art and Design, LSAD, that September, I was eighteen years old and seventeen stone two pounds. In other words I had achieved a personal goal; at long last I weighed less than my age. I certainly do not agree, now, with how I went about it but, at the same time, I remember my joy at getting on the scales and watching how the pounds were disappearing. Mam had to buy me new clothes because my usual wardrobe was too big for me – this was a brand new experience for me. It led to a newfound confidence in myself and, overall, I felt happier than I had in ages and ages.

No doubt thanks to my weight loss, I went out and got myself a job a few weeks before starting college, waiting on tables in Quenelle's, a popular restaurant in town. While the job was okay, in itself, I absolutely fell for the people I was working it. Here it was: a social life at last. I was the youngest there, but never felt left out in any way. In fact I had a ball as the people I worked with were so nice and for the first time in a long time I felt like I didn't have to worry about what other people thought of me or might say about me. My confidence was growing and the job really brought me out of myself. You cannot be shy and timid when dealing with the public. It was a far cry from the isolation I had experienced during the last year or two in school. The restaurant closed on Mondays so Sunday nights were our mad work nights out – which meant that when I turned up on a Monday morning for the LSAD introductory day for my course, I had to position myself as near as I could to the bin as I was a little worse for wear after a great night out.

CHAPTER THREE

MY WEIGHT BECOMES A PROBLEM

In September I started studying Fine Art and Design at LCAD and things were good. My diet had improved and I also joined a gym. My sister's boyfriend at the time was a body builder so I started training with him as I wanted to be able to lift weights properly. I was intent on turning my fat into muscle, as well as ridding myself of those man-boobs. I learned a lot, hanging out with other body builders at the gym, for instance I heard about the condition known as Body Dysmorphia. This is when a person is one hundred per cent convinced that they have a terrible flaw in their physical appearance. This 'flaw', as they see it, fills them with shame and they will literally spend hours focusing on it and how they can get rid of it. But, no matter what they do, in their eyes it never goes away.

I believe that I went through bouts of this, over the next few years, in that I couldn't see myself clearly. I got bigger and bigger, because I wanted to, believing that I was building muscle; I never saw that as well as all the muscle I was building, I was also getting fatter.

College did nothing for me in that art colleges are seen as 'arty farty', but to me it seemed more like a soft drugs scene. I was never into drugs or getting stoned and I didn't like the way some students put on airs, talking, dressing and acting like they were something special, something apart from the rest of us. It was just so false. Why would someone think they are more intelligent or more talented because they smoke joints? Maybe I wasn't complicated enough to study art. I got very bored listening to long, heated discussions on why an artist had painted something in a particular way ... you know, like why he put in a black dot when it wasn't necessary – was it his miserable childhood, his dark thoughts, a dejected pronouncement on his meaningless life? Ah, I hadn't the patience for it. I painted out of pure enjoyment, but all this stuff turned art into a chore, which horrified me. I dropped out, just stopped attending classes, and took to earning money instead, all the while keeping up my training regime at the gym. My parents were disappointed, they tried to get me to stay on, or even look for a trade to study, but I was adamant that I no longer wanted to be a student.

Just before Good Friday, in 1999, I started a new job as a bouncer. It paid more than the restaurant, a lot more; I could make 15 euro an hour for standing around talking to people. You could say that I was perfectly built to be a bouncer; I was about eighteen stone and over six feet tall. The job certainly had its share of perks, good money – and, for the most part it was easy money – I got see to some crazy stuff and make really good friends.

I must admit I really enjoyed being a bouncer. It's not for everybody.

If you get impatient with people who are drunk or take offence easily, this is not the job for you. Fortunately for me, it suited my particular temperament. Don't get me wrong, it was definitely not all sweetness and light. There were plenty of fights or near fights, instigated by bitter drunks who we could not let over the threshold, or else had to be escorted off the premises. As I began to get fatter again I was the easy target for any abuse that was going. However, I don't think it was the same as when I was being bullied in secondary school. For some reason I can mostly forgive someone for their antics when they are under the influence of alcohol. It would happen, from time to time, that someone, be they a girl or a bloke, who had given me dog's abuse on the Friday or Saturday night, would be mortified on bumping into me during the week, and profuse in their apologies. One red-faced girl admitted that she couldn't exactly remember what she had said to me, or the names she had called me, she just had this hazy memory of ranting abuse in my direction. Of course there were others who would pretend not to recognise me when they met me in the sober light of a Tuesday afternoon, but that just made me want to giggle.

The negative side of me looking the part of the bouncer was that it did not help to motivate me to lose weight or look after myself. I was surrounded by big men and it helped to be physically bigger than troublesome customers. Therefore it was a good thing to be the size that I was, I felt normal. In the mirror at the gym I could not appreciate that I was getting fatter, albeit slowly, as when the scales showed I was going up in weight I was so intent on making myself appear muscular that I felt it was muscle though was some was also fat. Working nights meant I was eating at the wrong time and it would not have been very healthy stuff either.

In March 2000 I started working for MCM Security and was posted to Brown Thomas in Limerick. It was here that one of the other security girls came to my attention. I hadn't had much success with women up to then. Like most people I suffered bouts of unrequited love and fancied women, but I just hadn't the confidence to make an effort, one way or another, until, that is, I met my new work colleague. Shelly was from Tipperary, had a bubbly personality and a cheeky glint in her eyes. We hit it off immediately, flirting with one another for weeks on end until finally we had our first kiss on 27 May; I can tell you this, not because I'm particularly romantic or very clever when it comes to remembering dates, but it was the day that Munster lost the Heineken Cup to Northampton, in Twickenham – now, that, I can never forget, but the kiss was pretty good.

We saw each other casually after that, for the next few months. I think I was aware that she was a lot more serious about us than I was and we finally parted some time later, in August of that year; while I liked her a lot I wasn't really interested in a relationship at the time. It was also about this time that I left my full-time position with MCM, and started my apprenticeship as an electrician, training under my uncle, Pat Scanlon. My life was busy. By day I was out on construction sites with Pat, Monday to Fridays, 8 – 5pm, including some Saturdays, while I still worked Sundays at Brown Thomas, and I also did a few nights bouncing for the Globe night club in Limerick. All in all I was working over sixty hours a week and training hard at the gym; as a result of being so busy I was always just eating on the go and just ate what was convenient. I did not have time to stop to think, or think about what I was putting in my mouth. Pat would cluck his disapproval when he saw me chomping my way through greasy breakfast rolls, but, not surprisingly, I was always tired and wanted to eat my way to energy, and if that meant a square meal of eggs, bacon and sausages squashed between two powdery sides of white roll, for the price of a pint, then so be it. Apart from those deadly, but delicious rolls, I was drinking one or two litre bottles of fizzy drinks on a daily basis, which was pure madness, though I did not know it at the time. They are addictive and full of sugar and I was relying on them to keep me awake for my sixty-odd-hour working week.

Now, I could be flippant and blame Weightwatchers for this. When you are working out your points system it is a lovely thing to be told that diet fizzy drinks contain no calories, I think it is fair to say I made what I wanted to of that piece of advice. Actually I can't really blame Weightwatchers, since I had always loved fizzy drinks. I preferred them to a chocolate bar any day of the week.

In late January 2001 Shelly and I began seeing one another again. This time it was different … I suppose I missed Shelly and from a chance meeting one night I knew I was ready. Within a short amount of time it got serious and I knew I had fallen in love with her. I was twenty-one stone when we met, so she only knew me as a big guy, I think it is important to say I am naturally a big guy at 6 ft 2 and I am broadly built so when I was twenty-one stone it was by no means a real issue at that stage and my weight never came between us. However, it became apparent that I would have to make changes, in order to fit her into my week, as well as work and training at the gym, so I cut back on my hours. And I began to put on more weight, just because

I was so happy with the relationship, it was another reason not to bother counting calories. Like most couples we started staying in and would either cook or get takeaway; like a lot of people who get very comfortable in a relationship and put on some weight, I got a little too comfortable.

In 2002 I went to Fás as part of my apprenticeship. This meant I was back sitting in a classroom for six months straight, which meant I was no longer getting any exercise on the construction sites. I think I put on about two stone over a few months of spending my week sitting behind a desk. For the first time in my life the physical affect of this was all too obvious to me, when, six months later, I returned to the construction site and found it increasingly difficult to work efficiently. I sweated profusely all day and then, when I was finished, I was absolutely shattered. My remedy for such exhaustion was the usual two litres of fizzy drink as I badly needed the caffeine and sugar boost. I was thirsty all the time, and never, ever, in a million years, would it have occurred to me to down two litres of water instead. It did frighten me to feel so unfit. I hadn't felt this bad in a long time, I did try to cut down on food on the go, but for some reason I just never really stopped and thought about the calories in fizzy drinks, my diet other than that wasn't that bad once we stopped having fast food on a Saturday night and I cut down on the breakfast rolls.

Shelly and I moved into an apartment together. It was my first time living away from home, and I loved us being together.

Out of contentment with Shelly, and silent misery at becoming a laughing stock once more, I turned to food with a vengeance. I put on even more weight, and guiltily watched Shelly put on weight too, as our social life became more and more about take-outs in front of the television. Neither of us was ever big into drinking, so once we got together our favourite way to spend an evening was in front of the TV set, watching our favourite programmes with a take-away. We wouldn't need a bottle of wine, just food, telly and us. It was the perfect Saturday night, especially after a long week, going between two jobs and training. All I wanted to do was relax. Then, because it was so enjoyable on Saturday night, we might do it again on Sunday. Sometimes, too impatient for Saturday, we'd get take-out on Friday. I was dragging her down, I only see that now, and I do have an enormous guilt over this. She did her best to get me back on track, and try to get me to eat properly, but I wouldn't listen to her.

I was still working very long hours, both as an electrician and on the doors as a bouncer. Financially, things were great. I would easily make €100 a night on the doors to supplement my apprentice wage, which wasn't great, so we didn't want for anything. But I realise now there was also a downside to this, in that I always had money in my pocket, money to eat on the go. Also living away from the family home for the first time I would be lying if a said I ate well; due to our hectic lives and Shelly working shifts, I ate more and more food on the go, sometimes a quick sandwich or cereal, other times a roll from a petrol station or even a takeaway. I did eat chocolate and sweets, but not too many. However, I was still drinking a lot of fizzy drinks probably two or maybe three litres a day at this stage and as you can expect my weight was just going up and up.

Life was good, as long as I could forget people looking at me on the street. Just as I had pretended to my parents, now I would put on a smiling face for my girlfriend, so she had no idea of the shame and humiliation that was becoming a regular part of my day. People must have thought I was blind as well as fat. Grown men and women would stare openly at me, not even looking away if I dared to meet the shocked expression on their faces.

I would love to say it didn't bother me but it did, not only was it affecting my day job, but at night it had turned to a nasty source of entertainment for drunk customers when they would be stopped or asked to leave and I would regularly get a lot of abuse about my weight. In the coming months it got worse and worse and it had a huge impact on me psychologically; it really got me down. I would come home from work at 3am absolutely drained and very angry at the abuse that was being hurled at me. No matter what time of the day it was, I would eat when I was down and at this stage I was down a lot as this abuse was becoming way too frequent and as a result my weight went up and up until I was around twenty-seven stone.

In all honesty, my eating habits were spiralling out of control and I was oblivious to it. What I wasn't oblivious to, though, was the looks I began getting on the street. It is hard to explain why I allowed myself to put on so much weight, without stopping to think about it. I was just busy earning a living, learning a trade and being happy in love. I ate when I was gloomy, when I was bored, and when I was happy. I blame the hours of bouncing that had me eating dinners in the middle of the night; that had to have been a factor. But it was those looks of disgust from passing strangers that made me gloomy and depressed. When I walked home from work I would see people in their cars staring at me, and I would pretend not to notice. It started to get in on me, not that

Shelly or my family would have been aware of this. I was too practised now, from my teens, in pretending everything was fine.

Shelly and I decided to buy a house, so that was something to work for, our future. Life continued on and, from to time, I would make a serious effort to lose weight. I was still training hard, four or five days a week, in the gym and the results were satisfying. I competed at both national at international levels, in powerlifting, and won a few gold medals.

Finally, I qualified as an electrician and decided to go into business with Spud, a guy I really liked, who had served his time with me. This was a good thing, and it wasn't a good thing. You see, Spud is skinny and is one of those people we all know who can eat anything and never put on a pound. He's always hungry. I don't know where he puts it, but any time he would go to the shop during work for junk food I found it impossible not to ask him to bring me back something too, usually fizzy drinks. It's just that we worked such long hours and were so busy, it was instantly habit-forming to say 'yes', when he'd ask me if I wanted anything.

We got engaged – Shelly and me, not Spud and me! The wedding date was set for 15 March 2007. It was like I was living in two worlds then. One world was Shelly and my family, which only ever made me very happy, my 'other life', while in most ways confined to the door where I worked, was starting to spread away from the door.

I went to work at night knowing that a night of abuse lay ahead. At times things happened by day too – not abuse, but it was fair to say I knew people looked at me and I knew what they were thinking. The result was that I wasn't happy, I was miserable. Why didn't I leave that job? Well, I was self-employed and we had bought a new house and were getting married and door work paid very well and I simply needed the money. I know a lot of bouncers and doormen who, like me, felt a little trapped – the money was too good, which made the job very hard to give up.

I was also a lot more aware of the way people would look and even stare at me; it did nothing to help my self-confidence, which added to my sense of worthlessness. Going out in public was becoming a problem for me, another one that I hid from everyone and probably myself too. I cannot remember exactly when it started, but I began to avoid places that were not 'safe' for me. What I mean is, that I only went where I was already known, which reduced the amount of attention I would get. I wasn't interesting in widening my small circle of friends; I was way too cynical and negative about being out in public.

As our wedding drew nearer I really wanted to lose weight, but I was so unmotivated. I just felt it was now too big a task, Shelly suggested we both go to Weightwatchers together in order to lose weight before the wedding. It was a futile effort as they didn't even have a scales that could weight me and so I quickly faded as I had no idea if the diet was bringing any results.

Just like with my Communion and Confirmation suits, my wedding suit would have to be specially made for me. It wasn't just that I was carrying so much weight. Thanks to my training, I had built up a fair amount of muscle and could find no jacket wide enough to stretch across my back and shoulders. As the big day approached I had no idea what weight I was as it had been a while since I had been able to weigh myself, but I am guessing I was thirty-one or thirty-two stone.

As always Shelly did her best to motivate me to do something about it, as did my family. But I think I felt I was beyond control and it was simply best not to think about it. I was so down in myself and relied on food too much to get through a bad day, plus it was taking everything I had to pretend I was fine.

I don't believe I was addicted to food. It was more, I feel, that I was in such a dark place that I turned to food for comfort. There cannot be many people reading this, no matter how thin they are, who haven't, after a row, or a bad day at work, enjoyed a snack purely because it made them feel just that bit better. I didn't open bottles of wine, smoke ten fags or sink six-packs of beer into me, I ate instead. When I felt crap, it made me feel better, for a while anyway. Thanks to this book I have had to look back and try, as best as I can, to understand my relationship with my eating habits. The best I can do is compare food to being a friend of mine. It was always there, sugar and salt, waiting to console me and provide me with bouts of comfort from the world outside and the depression I was brewing inside and I came to rely on it to make me feel better. However, it was not a true friend. It did not actually care for me; in fact it was the one causing me problems in the first place, making a fool out of me and sending me out on the streets to be laughed at. In other words, my good friend 'Food' was stabbing me in the back the whole time. Talk about a self-destructive relationship.

Shelly had started to ask me if I was okay, when I came home in the evenings, and I had to pretend I was just pissed off about work, or something general like that. There was no way I could tell her the truth, that I felt like a freak outside, since I was as sickened and embarrassed by it myself. A few months before the wedding, Mam suggested that I try to lose some weight. She was very concerned and told me, 'Gary, if you don't make the effort you're only going to get heavier and heavier, and then what? You could have a heart attack and die. Is that what you want?' Of course I told her 'no', but inside I swear I remember thinking to myself that I didn't really care anymore. Here I was, about to marry my best friend and I didn't care if I lived or died. I was scared but couldn't honestly believe it was possible to lose weight over the next few months. I had stopped believing that I could change. I felt defeated in every way. Worst of all I felt I had let everybody down.

In spite of everything the wedding was a wonderful day. We didn't go on a honeymoon immediately as we received the keys, at last, to our house and preferred to spend the money on furnishing it. I did feel a bit happier then. The future seemed brighter and I looked forward to this new life I had embarked on. I had my beautiful wife, our new home and we were planning on filling it with children. My sister had given birth to my god-daughter, Nicole, the previous year and I had completely fallen in love with her. When I was with her I forgot all about myself. She lit up my life in a whole new way; she was magical. Shelly and I couldn't wait to become parents ourselves and decided against waiting any longer.

So, things were relatively good. Spud and I were very busy at work, this was the height of the building boom and there was plenty of work. Spending time with my baby god-daughter proved just as comforting as eating food for comfort. A gurgling baby is the perfect antidote to a bad mood. Being around her made me more hopeful than I had been in a long, long time. It was a great reminder that I had a lot to be thankful for.

With this in mind I decided to go and speak to my doctor, at the time, explaining that I wanted to lose weight. He recommended a particular programme called Lipotrim, which I believe was commonly recommended by GPs, and had proved very effective for a lot of people who were serious about losing weight. It was a rather severe diet. Simply put, it involves not eating food. Instead, you drink three shakes a day, which contain all the minerals and vitamins you need. Meanwhile your body goes into a state called ketosis, whereby the body burns its own fat as fuel. Due to the severity of this plan, I went home to discuss it with Shelly, who decided that it would best if we did it together. Thanks to me, I feel, she had put on a few stone over the last couple of years so it made sense to support one another.

My God, but it wasn't easy. I hated the taste of the shakes which were very bland and, naturally, found it hard to stop wishing for favourites like fizzy drinks and starchy carbohydrates. Before starting the diet I managed to find a scales to weight me. I was thirty-four stone starting the Lipotrim diet. The next few weeks were bloody hard, although I did lose two stone. However, there was a flip side to this in that I developed respiratory problems. I began to experience such bad bouts of coughing that I ended up having panic attacks over not being able to catch my breath. I was really sick, spent a fortune on tablets, couldn't do anything much for weeks on end. I came off the diet due to being sick and, consequently, I put back on the two stone I had lost, and then some. On top of all that I felt very let down by my doctor. He didn't seem to want to discuss the problems I was having, from a diet that he had recommended to me. I decided I needed something else and was desperate enough to ask him to refer me to the national obesity clinic in Loughlinstown. He refused to give me one, telling me that all I needed to do was eat three healthy meals a day and take up walking. I couldn't believe what I was hearing. It must be difficult for some people to understand what it is like – as if it was as simple as that, me just merrily eating a good breakfast, lunch and dinner, and then going out for a stroll in the evenings. Walking was difficult for me, both physically and mentally, as I didn't want people looking at me. I left the doctor feeling very let down.

The year 2007 wasn't such a great one, thanks to the economic collapse. Every penny I had made over the years with my company, I had invested it in buying new equipment. I was determined to offer the best service I could to customers and wanted to stay ahead of the game. And it worked, our reputation spread and we were starting to win contracts from the bigger companies, who then started to go out of business, in twos and threes. I know it is a cliché, and one that has been said many, many times. Nevertheless, it certainly felt to me that the building boom crashed over night. One week there was work and the very next week it was all gone. All my hard work, and Spud's, was for nothing. Those days when we had worked twelve, fourteen hours, racing around to keep customers happy were a thing of the past. As they say, the bubble just burst. The only thing I had left from the company was debt … to the tune of €120,000. Everything we had was taken by the bank, all our expensive equipment was sold at a cut-rate price. Since I was the only one who owed a house it did seem like the banks focused especially on me.

I suppose the one good thing was that I knew it wasn't my fault. It is a blow to the confidence when something you build up, with everything you have, is taken away from you, but I couldn't blame myself for the Celtic Tiger running back to wherever it came from.

On the down side I was more and more down about myself, I had very much mastered hiding my pain, but I knew what people thought of me when they looked at me. This is actually something I have discussed with other overweight people. It is a common phenomenon that we like to call 'the look'. I cannot emphasise enough the devastating effect it can have on a person, when they are looked over, by a complete stranger, like they are nothing more than a large piece of dog shit. There is little or no compassion for people who over-eat. Alcoholics, anorexics, the crippled and intellectually challenged, most people can find pity in their hearts for these conditions, but for folk like me, all they have is horror and disgust. Maybe it is because gluttony is named as one of the seven deadly sins? You can see what they are thinking, *Gluttonous bastard; big fat, greedy pig*. It is horrible. This 'look' alone was the reason why I felt I could not face going to new places. As a result my world got very small.

Fortunately I had still kept up my bouncing work. I worked nightclubs and ended up as a security manager which paid good money but was very tough going. I've written before about having the right temperament for a bouncer but it to got to a stage where that wasn't enough. There were probably two reasons for that. Firstly I had gotten used to bouncing as a supplement to my wages, now I had to do it because the company was gone and I had a mortgage to pay. Secondly, my mood was low anyway, which no doubt made me more sensitive than usual. The job was tough, it is a big responsibility and you are constantly dealing with problems.

My duties included dealing with pretty much everything: hiring staff; organising training and rosters; dealing with the Gardaí; logging incidents; filing reports; checking CCTV recordings; investigating incidents. To be fair I was good at it. I obviously had a presence, thanks to my size, and I was not afraid to deal with people in a confident manner. Of course no matter how confident I behaved, it didn't mean I was relaxed. With certain types of customers you were always tense and ready for violence. Some of our customers were potentially dangerous folk and since I liked to lead by example, I would put myself on the frontline and stop them from coming into the club. Consequently, I was followed home more than once, with threats to 'get' me.

It was stressful. I would have preferred to walk away from it, but that wasn't an option. The hours were from 10pm to 3am, four nights a week, and when I got home I was so wired that I would stay up until six or seven in the morning. After dealing with particularly dodgy individuals, preventing entrance or barring them, some nights I sat there expecting my home to be attacked. Needless to say I was eating at night which would explain my not being able to sleep for hours on end.

I had thought I had a built a wall around me and could ignore the abuse, but when I look back now I cannot believe what I was allowing myself to deal with. The abuse was by far the worst it had ever been. On one occasion a disgruntled customer, a guy I refused entrance to, went away after calling me a lot of names. He returned, a few minutes later, with a bag of burgers he had bought specially and began throwing them at my feet, shouting, 'Go on, fat boy; eat them up! You know you want them. Eat them up, you big, fat fuck!' I had to stand there and pretend I was too tough to care.

The following year, Shelly and I finally managed to take our honeymoon. We left Ireland, in October, and flew out to Las Vegas first and then Mexico. I enjoyed Las Vegas, but I'm afraid I can't say the same about Mexico. The heat and the humidity were like nothing I had ever experienced before. The sweat was running off me, making me self-conscious about how that looked, and about being smelly. I felt like a stuffed pig. I felt like utter shit. Before I realised it, I was staying in the hotel room, not wanting to go outside and make a spectacle of myself.

CHAPTER FOUR

A DARK TIME

In 2009 Shelly and I were both made redundant from our jobs within four weeks of each another, I lost mine in early September, and she lost hers on 1 October. In hindsight I think, regarding my particular employment situation, this was a good thing. At the time it seemed like everything was coming down around me; nevertheless, losing my job meant that I was no longer working nights, taking dog's abuse from angry drunks nor eating at ridiculous hours. That was the good thing about losing my job. The bad thing was the obvious, as I am sure a lot of people will relate to, whether they are also fighting a battle with their body, or not.

Losing my job meant losing that small part of me that held my ebbing confidence and battered self-esteem. In my eyes everything that I had was going, bit by bit. I got very down, worried incessantly about money and was afraid for our future. I ate desperately, in search of some sort of solace and piled on more stones, making me feel worse than I already did. They were dark months, and I grew very bitter about myself and pretty much everything else. The bigger I got the more damaging it was in every way: physically, mentally and emotionally. But the saving grace, if you want to call it that, was that Shelly and I were not alone in this. A lot of friends and relatives were out of work. Still, I'm an old-fashioned guy and I couldn't stop thinking that I had let my wife down.

I am guessing that I was over thirty-five stone by now. You might read that figure and think to yourself, 'Wow, that's bloody heavy!' but you will probably not appreciate exactly what that meant, on a day-to-day basis. Let me try and show you.

This was my life for about twelve months or so. I would get up anytime between 9 and 10am. Shelly and I were in separate beds now because it was impossible for her to fit comfortably into our bed, due to my size, and even if there had been room I probably would have interrupted her night's sleep, as it was now normal for me to wake up, in dire pain, a couple of times a night, thanks to my habit of lying on my side, thereby crushing my own arm beneath my body. We were still being intimate, but the size of my penis had changed dramatically, as the rest of me got bigger. Of course it impacted on our love-making, which caused problems for both of us, on an emotional level. We so badly wanted a baby and it was becoming worrying that nothing was happening for us.

(In June 2009 Shelly and I decided to have our fertility tested. I thought that if only we could get pregnant, it would change everything, and we would have something truly wonderful to look forward to. I would have to guess that I was maybe thirty-five stone or more at this point. A guess is necessary since I couldn't weigh myself; I was too heavy for any scales I could get my hands on. So, my semen was tested and it was discovered that I was infertile. That day has got to be one of the worst days of my life. I tried to put a brave face on for Shelly, but the news devastated me. This was it; everything had been taken away from me now, including my future. I went home and I ate and I ate and I ate.)

Going to the bathroom was deeply upsetting. The toilet seat had to be removed to give me more room, and even then it was a struggle. I needed a special aid to wipe my bum and, because of my diet, I frequently had the runs or, at the very most, soft poo. There were also problems with plain old urinating, thanks to the amount of fat near my penis, which prevented me from aiming straight. To solve this problem I had taken to sitting down on the toilet to pee, or else I would have sprayed it all over the place.

Getting dressed could take a while. Putting on my socks required patience and diligence. I sweated heavily the whole time, so would have to apply talcum powder to my crotch, arm-pits and underneath the man-boobs, in an attempt to curtail both sweat and chafing. Once dressed, I went downstairs for a breakfast of Weetabix or porridge.

I pottered away the day. It can be done quite easily, if you don't stop to think about things too much. It was now imperative that I stayed indoors. Shelly did all the shopping because, apart from the gym, I loathed leaving the house, which meant leaving myself wide-open for abuse. At one stage, when I was still going outside, a guy actually took a picture of me on his phone. That might not sound like much, but think about it: you are walking along a street, minding your own business. Your confidence is low, you feel awful, you know you look bloody awful, yet you keep it together because you have to. Then it becomes apparent that you look way worse that you might ever have imagined, because it is not everyday that you stand out so much that someone feels obliged to whip out their mobile to take a photograph of you, because you are that bloody big he must be afraid that if he merely describes you to his mates they won't believe him. He needs actual proof of just how incredibly fat you are – I mean, I am.

God only knows how many people laughed over it.

When I did have to leave the house I would fret over needing to go to the loo. It was bad enough in my own house, but there was no way I would want to be caught out in town or wherever, and have to try to negotiate a public toilet, with a possible audience looking on. It was a constant worry until I discovered a resolution, in the form of popping a pill that would constipate me for a few hours, until I got home again.

Buying clothes became considerably easier as I just got stuff online, at huge expense, from special shops that catered for sizes like and 5x-large and 6x-large.

Shelly did all the housework since I wasn't able to do anything that required much effort. At that stage she was more like a carer than my wife. I really don't know why or how she stayed with me. I would not have blamed her in the slightest if she had have packed her bags and fled.

Lunchtime was a sandwich and a cup of tea, or maybe some fizzy drink.

I still managed to get to the gym, a few afternoons a week, to lift weights. Unfortunately one does not lose weight, or get fit, by lifting weight as it is about as static a sport you can get, apart from darts, I suppose. Not that I could have done much in the way of exercise, just walking a few steps made me out of breath. Actually my breathing was bad whether I was moving or not. My breath stank too.

We were also both trying hard to find work in a recession, filling out loads of applications for all sorts of jobs. I got called for a few interviews that led to nowhere. When I turned up I would always feel it would have been far better to stay at home. There was that 'look', over and over again, from the receptionist, from the other candidates and, lastly, from the interviewer. There was no way anyone was going to employ me.

At around 5pm Shelly would cook us a healthy dinner. We ate a lot of casseroles; they were cheap meals, apart from anything else. My portion was normal-sized. After my good dinner, however, was where I slid into temptation. Sitting in front of the television I would easily sip my way through two and four litres of fizzy drink, of an evening. There were also the nights that I ate a load of rubbish, alongside the fizzy drink.

So, that is what a normal day involved, physically at least. I felt rotten, like I was trapped by my own body. Nevertheless, the description does not represent what was going on with me mentally. And I can tell you now that I was in a dark, dark place. As I say, I stopped going out the front door, aside from my training sessions at the gym. Within the house I had stopped looking in the mirror. Actually, we only had the one mirror and that was in the bathroom that I never used. I simply could not bear to see myself. When I think about it, I didn't need a mirror to know how bad things were, hadn't I enough information from the people who stared at me in disgust.

My moods swung from anger to self-pity. For one thing I felt utterly isolated despite having the love of my wife and family. I was convinced that I couldn't talk to anyone about what was going on with me. Around my parents and siblings I still managed to put on a good face, and, of course, I doted on Nicole and enjoyed spending time with her. I watched programmes like *The Biggest Loser*, hoping to find someone I could relate to, who might understand how I felt, but that wasn't possible since I was so much bigger than any of the contestants.

Really, how did Shelly do it? I turned into a thoroughly negative person who loved nothing better than giving out about the world in general. Politics became my subject and I passionately denounced one and all from the couch, going on and on about the ills of our society. I moaned, I whined, I complained. I was irritable, short-tempered and, in short, must have been a complete nightmare to live with. I hated everyone – but not as much as I hated myself. While I never actually contemplated suicide, I did not care one little bit whether I lived or died. That was probably the crux of the matter; I literally stopped caring about myself.

I hit rock bottom. In a nutshell, Shelly and I were unemployed, with no sign of that changing for either of us. I was thirty-five stone, unable to walk much, enjoy the fresh air or leave the safety of my house for more than a couple of hours, owing to the fact that I couldn't, or wouldn't, use a public bathroom. Financially I was in just as bad shape. I owed money to the banks from my collapsed business and was infertile. Yeah, I hit rock bottom alright.

Is it true to say that when most people go through a long, bad patch, for whatever reason, that music becomes more important than usual?

Certain songs would speak to me. I am one of those people who like listening to music for the lyrics, the story of the song. Funnily enough, one of my favourite songs, from this time, was Christina Aguilera's ballad, 'Beautiful'. I could listen to that over and over again. Another song was 'God and Satan' by Biffy Clyro, the Scottish rock band. When I listened to the words, I found them both dark and comforting, and I would tell Shelly that I felt they aptly described the pair of us. I'm not so sure she found that such a comforting thought, as some of the words are about a guy acknowledging how his lover sticks around even though he knows he makes her miserable, and may even ruin her life.

However, the most important song for me, by far, was Nick Cave's 'Into My Arms'. As soon as I heard this song I thought of Shelly. When I would sing along to it, I would actually be singing it to her. The lyrics describe how much she means to me. Throughout it all, she was the bright light in my life. I had loved her for years, even when I'm sure she thought I was only thinking about myself and my problems. The worst thing of all is believing that I had brought her pain when I should have only brought her joy and protection from anything that might upset her. This song says it perfectly for me, it has become 'our' song, so much so that I told Shelly I wanted it played at my funeral. A funeral I had spent too much time thinking about, frequently sure it would be happening sooner rather than later. My idea was that if Shelly heard this song, after I died, she would know it was me, that I would always be near her and waiting for her, no matter what.

Somebody had to take a first step, and that somebody was Shelly. After sending out umpteen job applications, and getting nowhere, she made the brave decision to go back to college. In September 2010 she enrolled as a mature student, to do a degree in Business, to major in Human Relations, in the University of Limerick. I was so proud of her, and doubly ashamed of spending my days, Monday to Friday, sitting in the house, unable to face the world, out of pure fear, waiting for her to come home to me. What kind of a husband was I? What kind of a life was I giving her?

It was during one of long, dark days of doing very little, that it occurred to me that I owed it to her; I owed it to Shelly to try again.

So, this was it. I was going to lose weight, but how much did I need to lose? I had no idea how big I was, no ordinary scale could have withstood my standing on it. I needed to know the exact figure because I needed to set a goal.

For the last couple of years I was a regular listener to the *Ray D'Arcy Show*. When I worked as an electrician we always had the radio on, for either Ray or Gerry Ryan. Initially, as far as I was concerned, the radio was just background noise, on an already noisy work site, but then I found myself listening to Ray, putting on his show whether I was at work or not. The radio is great company. I felt like I knew Ray and his crew about as well as I knew the guys I worked with. On Fridays there was this thing, where if someone had a problem they would write into the show and Ray would try to help them with it. Little did I know how important that was about to become to me.

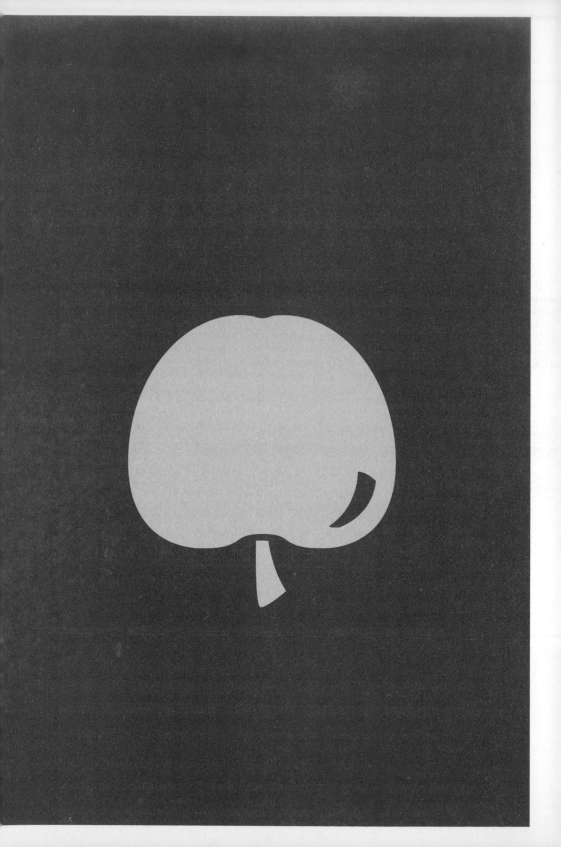

PART TWO

CHAPTER FIVE

'THE FIRST YEAR OF THE REST OF MY LIFE'

Sometime in October 2010 just after Shelly started in the University of Limerick as a mature student I found myself sitting in my mother's kitchen one afternoon having a heart to heart with Mam about my weight. Shelly and I had really been through the mill, but her going back to college really made me look at myself. She was willing to go back to college in order to give us a better future and in some ways I felt almost guilty; *I* should be the one taking such steps. It's not that I am a chauvinist, but maybe I'm a typical man – I like to think it's my job to protect Shelly and give her the life she deserves so, when it was her taking the first steps I found myself feeling like I had to step up and do the same, but what could I do?

As we sat chatting, I remember my mother asking me about my weight and for the first time ever I didn't just nod and agree, I actually listened. We had a chat, even a cry, and I came away knowing what I could do to help us. It didn't quite happen straight away, but a few days later I found myself talking to my cousin John Kirwan. John was in my class in CBS. He left in Fifth Year and in some ways I always felt that after John left the bullying started, as up until that he would stand up for me. John and I are roughly the same age and as we stood talking that day I listened intently as John, who has a lot of health problems, spoke about being sick and how it affected him and, in particular, his kids. I walked away thinking, 'John would do anything in the world to be better and here I am. I can do this if I really try.'

So I decided this was it; I was going to do it. I don't think I really stopped to consider how, but I was going to. The first thing I needed was a weighing scales, but with money being so tight I really felt under pressure. My mother said, 'Well, if that's all that's holding you back I will get it for you.' So I went in search of a scales so I could at least find out my exact weight and monitor it. That search was the start of an amazing journey.

I think I will always remember January 2011 as a huge turning point; it was when I took what turned out to be a life-changing decision – the decision to email 'Fix it Friday'. The next twelve months were in some ways a whirlwind and in some ways a slog, and I wanted to remember every minute of it, so on the advice of my brother Darren and his wife Eadoine – who said I could use it to track the diet and myself, allowing me to appreciate the changes, however minor, that I hoped would come about – I reluctantly decided to keep a diary. I'm going to quote from it extensively in this section and you'll see that I had ups and down, days of elation and days when I almost despaired. One thing that's very clear, though, is that sending that email into Ray

D'Arcy's show was inspired. All I wanted was something big enough to weigh myself on; I had no idea and no expectations beyond that. As is obvious from my diary, they gave me a great deal more than weighing scales.

The year began with the email to the *Ray D'Arcy Show*, which was read out to the nation on 14 January. I needed a special weighing scales and had been trying to order one from America, but they didn't deliver outside America – I was so frustrated. What kind of company, in this day and age, does not deliver internationally? I was at the end of my tether, when I thought of 'Fix it Friday'. I used Shelly's name for the email so no one would cop it was me as I was so embarrassed about what my life had become.

Dear Ray, Jenny and Team,

My husband is a big guy (we think 35+ stone) and the problem is that we can't find a scale that will weigh him accurately. We live in Limerick and we need to find a scale, as soon as possible, preferably in Limerick, that we can use once a week, or we can buy one although we can't afford to go over €150, and, so far, they are proving to be a lot more expensive than this.

My husband has been working really hard lately to lose the weight. I think he has lost a few stone already, but not knowing for definite is really affecting him as it is very hard to remain focused, and I don't want him to give up. I know that if we find a scale and he can start weighing himself regularly, it will really help motivate him.

So, please guys, I really need your help. This is literally life and death, we have tried Weightwatchers and lots of other places, but nobody has a scale that big. There is one in Cork, but we couldn't afford to travel there every week.

I really hope you can help us.

Regards,

Shelly

When I told her what I'd done, Shelly thought sending the email was a good idea, which was a relief, as I wasn't sure how she would feel about it. I had to go out and told her to listen to the *Ray D'Arcy Show* for me, in case I missed the 'Fix It' segment. However, as I was driving out of our estate, Ray read out my request. Yikes! My heart was in my mouth.

Bloody hell! I couldn't believe the response it got. The show received lots of emails and phone calls, but the listeners didn't really understand what I was after – the scales had to be calibrated so that it could give me an accurate reading of my weight. All the suggestions were off the mark, or involved something I had already tried. It was frustrating that, after all that, I was still in the same position. I rang Shelly and asked her to send a second email explaining the actual problem about the scales, and about it needing to be calibrated. In other words, it has to be 100 per cent accurate and checked regularly to maintain that standard.

I remember this like it was yesterday, I was standing in Moloney's Yard, Limerick, when suddenly, my phone rang; it was Siobhan Hogan, one of the researchers, from the *Ray D'Arcy Show*, needing me to explain exactly what I was looking for. I was really surprised. She was so easy to talk to and put me at my ease immediately. They wanted to get the right information out before the show ended. I was impressed with their eagerness to help and really wanted to believe that they could help me.

My plan to remain anonymous didn't work, however. My phone was beeping away all day with text messages, asking if that was about me on the radio. At around 12pm when the show ended my heart sank a little as they still had no definitive answer and so I decided I would just keep looking, I wasn't willing to give up. However, Siobhan rang back, about 1pm, to tell me that they thought they had found the correct scales! We chatted for a while and then she asked me if I would consider going onto the show to talk about my weight and myself. I was a bit taken aback, but said I would. She told me to think about it and that she'd call back later. When I got home I told Shelly, who was also taken aback. We hadn't expected this but, if it meant I could get a scales to help me, then it would be worth it.

Siobhan rang about 3pm with the brilliant news that they had found the right scales, though she was a bit vague about the details; a company was going to lend me a scales for a few months. I was over the moon. She asked me plenty more questions about myself, including if there was anything I would not be comfortable talking about on air. I could hardly believe I was having this conversation. So, we made a date for me to go up to Dublin to their studio on Monday morning, where Ray would interview me about my weight-related problems.

Once we hung up on one another I was suddenly filled with doubt, I was so determined to get the scales I never stopped to think about what they were asking me to do. What in God's name had I just agreed to? Did I really want to do this? Millions of thoughts jammed in my head and the most positive one was that if I went ahead, went public, it would force me to stick to the diet or else I would look like an ape, after all this fuss and at least I would know my weight one way or another no matter how bad it was.

Later that day, I met up with a friend of mine, Mike, who lives in our estate. He asked me about exercising and whether I could take up walking. He was very understanding when I explained about the difficulties with my knees, agreeing that swimming would be better for now. However, I had to admit that I did not have the money to join a gym. Without saying anything to me he went off and approached the Manager of JJB's, the local gym, who immediately offered me three months membership for free. Talk about a light at the end of the tunnel, I couldn't thank him, or the manager, enough.

That same evening, my sister called over with Nicole, and when I told her about Monday she was immediately nervous, asking me, 'Are you sure you want to be talking about your weight on the radio, telling everyone your business?' At first I was a bit annoyed, but then I had to thank her (silently, in my head!), because she instantly made me determined to go ahead with it. I know she was worried about me, what if they made a fool of me? What if the listeners were cruel, but her concern was actually reassuring – I knew my family had my back. At the very worst I was going to find out my exact weight at last. Anything else would be a bonus.

Shelly and I had a good talk. I told her that it had felt really good to be talking about the situation with Siobhan. It was the first time that I had opened up to anyone about what had been going on and it had felt amazing to be so open and not be judged

I decided that I needed to talk to my entire family before going on the radio on Monday; I'd hidden a lot of crap from them, which I knew would have to come out, and I didn't want them hearing it for the first time, on the radio, along with the rest of the nation.

On Saturday morning I went to my parents' house and was relieved to find my sister and one of my brothers there with my dad, but my mother was out. I started by confessing that Shelly and I couldn't have children because of my weight, and was shocked to see my dad cry a little. We spoke a bit about going on the radio on Monday and it felt really good to be sharing with them about my weight and the problems it was causing me in my life.

I was feeling really, really nervous about Monday, but I just tried to concentrate on the fact that I'd be getting the scales. Some of my fear had to do with finally being weighed. Shelly thought I could be about thirty-five stone, while I had a feeling that I could be a bit more than that, maybe thirty-six or thirty-seven stone, at the very worst.

Shelly offered to come with me, but I said no as she would have to miss a day of college; however, this was just an excuse. I just thought I'd be better going alone, as God knows what kind of state I'd be in. Mike offered too and I was about to say 'no' to him, but then I reckoned that he might be a good distraction, as he has a very light-hearted character. So, I arranged to meet him in Portroe at 7.30am, on Monday morning.

On the morning of Monday 17 January I woke up at 5am, terrified. How in the name of God was I going to go through with this? I really wanted the scales, but I was starting to panic over what Ray might ask me. After several more thoughts like this, I got up, trying to ignore the butterflies in my stomach.

After picking up Mike we got a flat tyre. My first thought was: *Grand, I might not make it to Dublin in time.* My second thought was: *I need those bloody scales though!* We got the wheel changed and were back on track, reaching Dublin with thirty minutes to spare. I did my best to relax, while Mike kept things cheerful. In fact I didn't feel too bad, at this point. This feeling didn't last. About ten minutes before I was due at the Today FM studios, I succumbed to terror once more. My heart was racing; I was covered in sweat while my throat was bone dry. The time was trickling by, ever so slowly, ironically giving me plenty of time to work myself up into a right state. Finally, it was time to get out of the car and head into Marconi House.

The thing I remember about walking into the Today FM reception area is the glass panels on the floor; I was afraid to walk on them for fear I would crack them. Siobhan Hogan met us at the reception desk, we spoke for a minute and then she brought us down to the studio. I think I started to feel a little less panicked once I was actually there. From then on my first time at the studio was a bit of blur. Everything seemed to happen at once. I met Ray, Will and Mairead, quite literally a couple of minutes before I went on air. It was a light chat that never got very personal, for which I was very grateful.

Things got a bit difficult when I was finally weighed: 577 pounds, or 41.3 stone. This was even worse than I had anticipated. Jesus Christ! I was over fucking forty-one stone. Ray read out the number while I remained speechless, panic building up inside of me because I knew I was on the verge of tears, I bit hard on my lip to try and stop myself from crying. I just wished the ground would open up and swallow me. It was one of those unforgettable moments that will haunt me forever. How did this happen? No, how could I have allowed this to happen? What the fuck had I done to myself? I am pretty sure that everyone, including Ray, could see the shock and mortification on my face. There was an awkward silence, because, really, what could anyone have said at a moment like that?

Ray finished off the interview with some comments and texts from the listeners, which were surprisingly supportive. Ray wished me well and I left the studio with the scales never expecting to return.

On the drive home, Mike told me that Siobhan had said that they might have me back on the show, over the coming months, because they were thinking that they might want to keep track of my progress and see if they could help me further. Convinced he had misunderstood her, I dismissed this. Nobody had said anything to me.

When I got home, I was gobsmacked. The amount of messages, both on Facebook – from one-liners wishing me luck, to more detailed emails, asking how I was and what I was going to do – and to my phone was overwhelming.

I listened back to the show and was happy enough with how I came across, apart from the weighing-in bit. It was a spooky coincidence when I heard the song Ray played just before I came on, Nick Cave's 'Into My Arms'.

Extracts from my diary show how I was feeling at the time.

Monday 17 January:

What a weird Monday it has been. I'm not sure what I think. I suppose I should be a bit excited over the fact that this is a new beginning for me, after the last few years of feeling trapped. Yet, tonight, as I sit here, writing this, I mostly just feel sickened with shame at finding out that I weigh over forty-one stone.

I woke up on the morning of Tuesday, 18 January 2011 determined to change my life. I decided to join a gym so that I could swim there every morning. I also planned to eliminate all the crap from my diet: fizzy drinks, fast food, sugary food and bread, to mention the obvious ones. In their place I began to eat brown rice, chicken and vegetables twice a day, with little knowledge behind this decision. There was no great plan in my head; these were merely the necessary first steps. It probably helped that I am a stubborn person. This became my strength, I made up my mind to change and nothing was going to stop me from doing that. What I didn't realise, however, was how much help I was going to get from so many sources.

Tuesday 18 January:

Well, today was the start of the rest of my life. I gathered my courage to go swimming. Mike said he'd come with me. Fair play to him! In truth I had been dreading it. Walking along the street, fully dressed, was difficult enough. I was determined, however, that nothing was going to stop me, neither my fears nor the looks I knew I was going to receive. As soon as I was in my swimming trunks I made my way to the water as fast I could, concentrating only on the ground in front of me. I have to say that I enjoyed it. It felt good to be swimming again. Of course, I hated the getting in and out, I was so paranoid about people staring at me, but I was thrilled I had done it. To be honest, I felt I had done something brave, which was a new feeling for me.

As far as I am concerned, this is it now. I am going to sort out my mess for me and for Shelly. I don't care what I have to do;

this is not going to be my life anymore. It is a bit of a surprise to discover that I feel really liberated after yesterday. I had been expecting to receive some negativity, especially after I was weighed, but all I got were positive messages from well wishers, friends and strangers.

Thursday, 20 January:

I went swimming again today and it was a bit easier than yesterday. I still got into the pool as quickly as I could to escape being stared at, but it was a lot quieter which was great.

People are asking me how much weight I want to lose. I suppose I hope to get around the twenty stone mark, but it's not just about losing weight. There is a lot of bullshit that I'm hoping to make disappear. To help myself focus I am going to make out two lists. Most things will be pretty ordinary for most people, but they are all hugely important to me.

I want to be able to:

Have children

Use a seatbelt in a car

Shop for clothes in a normal shop, like Penneys, Dunnes etc.

Walk up the stairs and not be out of breath

Tie my shoe laces without discomfort or difficulty

Use a standard public toilet

Sit in a seat in Thomond Park without being afraid I won't fit (or break it)

Sit in any seat anywhere and not be afraid that I will break it or that I won't fit

Cycle – it must be ten years since I've been on a bicycle

Travel without fear and anxiety

Go out and have fun

Take Shelly dancing, because we never properly danced at our
wedding

Travel in comfort on a plane

I don't want to be:

Afraid of large crowds and wide open spaces

Stared at

Constantly aware that people are looking at me in disgust

Ashamed

On the defensive

The way I am now

Wow, that really puts things into perspective. I feel sick.

I had to go downstairs, after writing out the above, and cry my
eyes out. The last couple of days have been intense so I suppose it
was only natural that I needed to release my emotions.

Yikes! I have just found out that I'm in tomorrow's **Limerick
Leader,** even after saying that I did not want to do an interview.

Friday 21 January:

I feel as if the weighing scale calls to me in the mornings. I can't
seem to stop weighing myself.

Well, I'm on the cover of the **Limerick Leader,** which was a bit of
a shock. I certainly never saw this happening a couple of months
ago!

Will Hanafin rang me, today, from Today FM. He says that the station is looking into how they can best help me, and, as a starting point, wonder if I would go and see a physiologist. So I'm heading to Dun Laoghaire, on Monday to see a guy they recommended. I have no idea what to expect.

Saturday 22 January:

Had a bad start to the day when, on waking up, I felt utterly drained of energy. I wonder if it's my diet. I have eliminated all bread, potatoes, white rice, pasta and all rubbish food. Greasy breakfast rolls are now a thing of the past; instead I have porridge without sugar.

I had to force myself to go swimming and I'm very relieved that I did. This guy approached me and asked if I was the fellow off the radio. It was a strange experience, but he was really friendly and supportive, and made me feel a lot more positive than when I had arrived at the pool.

I am starting to really enjoy the swimming. There is something very therapeutic about it. I swim forty lengths, at my own pace, and, as I swim, I am able to think about things. I find myself wondering how this big desire for change came about. It seems so sudden. One day I'm lying on the couch, in front of day-time television, too scared to leave the house – and now I'm on the radio, in the local paper and swimming every single day. It is strange how things work out.

Monday 24 January: (Weight: 566lbs)

I have lost 11lbs, in just one week! What a thrill it was to stand on the scales. It put me in a great mood and I headed off early, to the gym. When I came home I got ready for Dublin. I brought my own lunch of a couple of chicken breasts and a bottle of water. So long to the rolls I would usually buy at a petrol station, along the way.

As I drove I fretted over my appointment with the physiologist, wondering what he would ask me about. A small part of me wondered that maybe if I said something wrong to him that Today FM might not want to help me anymore.

I needn't have worried. All he wanted me to do was fill out three books of questions, about four hundred questions in total, and, to be honest, a lot of them felt like they were the same question asked in twenty different ways. I answered them as best I could, gave the books to the doctor who wished me well and said he would send on his report as soon as it was done.

Whatever about the report, I was feeling really happy, and was not tempted to stop at a garage to buy something to supplement my meagre lunch. When I got home Shelly and Mam were full of questions too, that I answered as best as I could.

Tuesday 25 January:

That was a strange experience yesterday. I had thought that the doctor would unlock something inside me, or give me some answers himself. I suppose I'll just have to wait and see what comes out of it.

Okay! My first goal is going to be this: if the Ray D'Arcy Show asks me back, I want to have lost two or three stone, at least. Will vaguely mentioned having me back but I was too shy to push him on this. In any case, if I am not asked back, I'm quite happy to do this myself. I'll just continue on with the diet and the exercise, though I know I will need to get help, at some stage, about what I'm doing. In the meantime, as long as I'm losing weight, that is all that matters.

Thursday 27 January:

I am like a bear with a sore head today. I don't know what is wrong but I feel like complete shit, and have, so far, bit the head off both Shelly and Mike for no real reason. This has been the toughest day yet. I have a blinding headache, since first thing this morning, and my body just feels crap!

Friday 28 January:

I cannot understand it. I had a really good swim this morning which made no difference to my mood. I just feel low and depressed in myself. It is so hard to keep motivated when I feel this shit.

Saturday 29 January:

Another shit day! I'm like an anti-Christ and I don't know why. If I keep this up Shelly will leave me. I didn't even bother going swimming, which is bad, and then I felt like a shit for missing it.

Sunday 30 January:

I'm not even going to bother writing about today, it was that bad!

I didn't know or recognise this at the time, but this feeling, which lasted a few weeks, was actually sugar withdrawal; going from so much sugar to no sugar my body had pretty severe withdrawal, which had both physical and mental effects on me.

Monday 31 January: (weight: 554lbs)

I lost ten pounds in weight last week, which is great, but doesn't help me to feel any better in myself. At least I went swimming, despite my body feeling lethargic. Okay, I know my weight is a factor but I really don't think I should be feeling this tired. Should I go and see a doctor?

I spent some time today researching diet information on the internet. Well, not so much diet as nutrition. However, I wasn't too sure what I was after and found it all a bit overwhelming.

Right, decision made! If I'm still feeling this bad tomorrow I'm going to go see a doctor. The exhaustion is hampering my efforts to do more exercise. I went into the gym this morning after my swim, and could hardly move. I am wondering if it is anything to do with the fact that I cut out all carbohydrates.

Friday 4 February:

I saw the doctor on Wednesday. He took my bloods to have them tested. All I can do is wait to see what comes back.

Today was another shitty day. Thank goodness I managed to go swimming but it took every bit of energy I had.

Jenny Kelly, from Today FM, rang me in the afternoon. It was my first time to talk to her and I must say she was lovely, very warm and supportive of what I was doing. Her call cheered me up, which was badly needed, as I was feeling so low again. She asked me if I'd come on the show again, next week, saying they had found something to help, but she wouldn't tell me what. It was wonderful to hear that they are still interested in me. For the first time in a while I felt better in my head, despite my tiredness. I'm really looking forward to seeing them all again.

Monday 14 February: (weight: 544lbs)

Happy Valentines Day! I have lost thirty-three pounds to date, and celebrated by doing a bit of DIY painting in the house. This is a big achievement! A few weeks ago I would not have been capable of doing anything like this. Shelly would have had to do it while I watched from the couch. I wasn't out of breath while I was working and didn't even feel wrecked after it.

Despite some ups and downs, my weight loss was off to a good start and I was determined to keep it up, no matter how hard it was. On Wednesday 16 February, I was due back in Dublin for an appearance on the *Ray D'Arcy Show*. I brought the scales in with me and, at the reception desk I had one of my first encounters with a listener; a guy came up and said 'hello' to me, adding that he had been following me on the show and wanted to wish me all the best. I hadn't a clue who he was, but it was nice of him to say that. This kind of thing was to happen more and more as the months went on, and it was a great help and encouragement to me, to know people were following my journey and wishing me well. Jenny came down to meet me. She was as friendly as she had been on the phone, while I was a bit shy and awkward, and led the way to Ray's studio.

This time I was a lot more relaxed for the interview, though I shocked Ray when I described how I would constipate myself if I had to go on a long journey, just so I would not have to face a public toilet. They want me to do join the Motivation Weight Management Clinic. I initially said 'no' on air when Ray mentioned it. I had contacted them about two years ago and thought they seemed expensive. Ray said we would discuss it off air, and after he convinced me to give them a try, adding that if I later felt it wasn't for me, then we could explore other options.

After my interview I returned to my car, and was busy putting the scales in the boot, when a truck pulled up, blocking the entire street, and the driver, with the thickest Dublin accent ever, roared out at me, 'Fair play to ya, buddy! You're doing great. Keep it up!' It made me smile.

Thursday 17 February:

I got a phone call from TV3 today! **The Midweek Show** wants me to come on and talk about my story. Panicking slightly, I told them that they would have to talk to the Ray D'Arcy Show. Speaking on the radio is one thing, television is something different altogether.

I was thrown when Jenny rang and said it was grand for me to do **The Midweek Show**, if I wanted to. What to do? I presumed that Today FM would say no, freeing me from having to make the decision. Well, TV3 will have to wait until tomorrow; I need time to think about this. Jesus!

I had been thinking about Ray's suggestion about Motivation Weight Management Clinic, and in February, I decided to go with them, I was still sceptical, but I decided I needed to go in with an open mind and I also felt that I didn't want to say 'no' to the first thing Today FM suggested. Following a battery of tests, I was put on a ketosis diet, a very severe diet that I don't mind saying I struggled with. But then any diet is hard, isn't it? Up to this point I had relied on this friend of mine – food – to get me through the bad patches, which were numerous, thanks, ironically enough, to my choice of friend. Now I had to cut myself lose from 'his' grip and do my best to ignore blatant yearnings for fizzy drinks. I was hungry for days and weeks on end, and perhaps this is something that I haven't dealt with on Ray's show – just exactly how hard it was. It is not that I was holding back, but I had decided not to be openly negative about my new life in case it affected my drive to keep going forward. I felt that if I started talking about all the drawbacks and negative parts of the diet, I would become bogged down by these, whereas if I focused on the positives I would keep focused on all the good parts of the diet. This worked really well, but it was still very, very hard. It was all about protecting me, and my new self that was trying to emerge out of forty-one stone. However, there was no arguing with the fact that on this diet I began to lose weight and it felt bloody brilliant.

In the early days I admit to being slightly addicted to weighing myself. Once Today FM got me those scales and once I saw I was losing pounds it was hard not to keep checking my weight: clothes on, clothes off, in the morning, in the evening, and so on. Although I am sure that this is a common feature regarding dieting and weight loss. And you can see from the diary that there were bad days. My mood would dip even though I might have lost a few pounds that week. I could still get depressed, but again, this is a normal part of any transformation process, when you are forced – frequently – to defend your decision to yourself.

<u>Friday 18 February:</u>

Paul, from the Motivation Clinic, rang today and talked me through the diet. It is not as scary as I thought it was going to be, so I'm going to give it a go. I had a second phone call from Motivation, later on, from a girl who introduced herself as Siobhan; she has been chosen to work with me. Fortunately I liked the sound of her. She seems to understand where I'm coming from. So, we're meeting up on Tuesday morning at 10am.

Big announcement: I am going to do the TV3 show. I mean, I will be very, very scared but I was thinking that it would be a chance to show people that there is more to me than fat. If people understand what it is like, it just might cut down on the looks of disgust that are fired at large people on the street.

I had a bit of a quiet day. Sometimes I feel a million, billion miles from where I want to be. While some of the things on my list will be achievable, I think the more difficult ones are under the heading of what 'I don't want to be'. My head is a bit raw, from having, I suppose, to think and talk about stuff that I never would. I was explaining this to Dad earlier. The more I talk about my life, the more I realise just how shit it is.

<u>Monday 21 February: Week 6 (weight: 542lbs)</u>

I have only lost 2lbs last week, and I'm not sure why. It is a bit of
a blow. All in all, I have lost two and a half stone, though I can't
see it myself. I guess I need to keep my head down this week and
work extra hard. Now that I think about it, I wonder if it could
be because I ate breaded fish a few times last week. To be fair, I
had no choice since I didn't have the money for fresh fish. Being
unemployed sucks!

    Met the **Midweek** crew today: Ciara, the presenter and Rob, the
cameraman. They arrived down about 11am and we filmed for
almost three hours. Ciara put me at ease and I actually enjoyed it.

<u>Tuesday 22 February:</u>

I met with Siobhan in Motivation today. We talked for two hours
or so, and covered just about everything I wanted to. She's really
nice and it is so bloody good to be able to talk to someone who
has been through it all, and knows what it's like. The diet is a bit
severe, which worries me, but if it works, it will be worth it. It is
a ketosis diet, high in protein with absolutely no carbohydrates
or sugars. This way my body will only consume protein and burn
my fat for fuel. Due to the severity of the diet, I can only stay on
it for a year. I suppose I should admit that this type of diet was
what my old doctor recommended, but at least I will have Siobhan
to consult with and, also, they will weigh me every week which is
great motivation in itself, no pun intended!

    It was gas. Danielle, their receptionist, is tall and thin, and I
couldn't believe it when she pulled out a photograph of herself,

before she lost four stone. I would not have recognised her as being the same girl.

Wednesday, 23 February:

I was supposed to start the Motivation Diet today but because I was heading to Dublin, for TV3, I decided to put it off until tomorrow. Siobhan gave me lots of information that I still have to read and I will also have to go and buy the food on the sheets. That is another reason I put it off, I had no money today!

Ciara from TV3 rang to tell me that **The Sun** newspaper wanted to send out a journalist and photographer to do a story on me, but I said no.

I left for Dublin at about 3pm, picked up Rob (my brother) along the way and we went to the Red Cow for a bite to eat. At 7pm we headed to the studios. I was very nervous, and very glad that Rob was with me. He had a great laugh when I was having my face caked up for the cameras. We sat in the corridor for an hour, waiting to be called, and were as giddy as school-boys.

Ciara came down and explained how it was going to go, and then the presenter, Sarah, came out to introduce herself.

Finally it was time to sit in front of the cameras. Actually I think the interview went very well, and felt happy enough after it, plus the relief of having got through it was immense.

We belted home to watch it with my parents, and when it came on, my phone went mad with texts and Facebook notifications.

I came back here and was relaxing on the couch, watching Vincent Brown, when he does a round-up of tomorrow's newspapers and guess who is in **The Sun**? The heading is awful, 'I Want To Be Big Daddy!' I felt sick. What on earth could they have written about me, without talking to me? WTF!

Thursday 24 February:

I didn't sleep well last night, thanks to the fright I got, watching Vincent Brown!

At 8am I ran out and got the paper. My fingers were shaking as I opened it up, but the article wasn't that bad at all. I just hate the tabloid heading that they used, that's not what I'm about at all.

Finally started the Motivation Diet today, and feel I can eat practically nothing.

This is one of my diet sheets:

7am   Breakfast protein bar

11am   protein drink or bar

1pm   Lunch: chicken, broccoli, cauliflower, no sauces

4pm   protein drink

7pm   Dinner: chicken or white fish, cauliflower, broccoli, no
         sauces

8-9pm   protein bar

Friday 25 February:

This diet is awful, and it's only the second day.

Got home at 8pm to find Shelly, out the front, talking to Adam, our neighbour. When she came in she told me he thought I was doing great, and said fair play to me. This is what I need to hear, positive support. I'm doing my best to stay away from any negativity, any doubt that I won't, or can't lose twenty stone over the next year.

Sunday 27 February:

This morning I asked Shelly to throw me down a t-shirt. She picked my orange animal one, which I hadn't worn in a while because it got so tight. Well, today it was fairly loose, and did that feel good!

I am so, so, so, so, so, so, hungry! God! This has been a shit week. Thank God for sugar-free jelly, that's all I can say.

Monday 28 February: (Week Seven) (weight: 528lbs)

In total I am down three and a half stone/forty-nine pounds, and I am very happy with that.

It was another hard day on the diet, especially around 6pm when I could not stop thinking about food. Of course it doesn't help that the smell of freshly-baked bread is all around, thanks to our proximity to a Tesco Express. If I had to name one food that I miss the most it would have to be bread: all bread; any types of bread. With these pleasant thoughts in mind I had to make do with feasting on sugar-free jelly.

I was wondering if I am going through the menopause. I cried like a baby tonight, while watching the final show of **The Biggest Loser**. I felt deliriously happy for the contestants, Claire, Will and Paddy, because they got their lives back, at last. I cannot wait to get to that point, they are so lucky.

Shelly got some garlic and onion salt today, which made a huge difference to my dinner. Dare I say it, it was almost nice.

Tuesday 1 March:

The weather was magnificent today. When the sun is shining
and the sky is clear blue you can't help but feel good. However,
the pool was freezing, besides which I got really pissed off when
swimming this morning. Some people are so rude, cutting into my
lane and throwing me off balance, when they can clearly see I am
doing lengths.

At this stage, I was still finding the Motivation diet very tough, and
I found the press attention very strange. Why was anybody interested
in my story? I had come from such a dark place I could not help but
be a little guarded.

It was around this time that I began to feel my perception of myself
changing; I felt that I no longer wasted time talking about doing
something, rather I had become a 'do-er'. If I wanted change, I had to
do my best to make it happen. The beginning of change in my sense of
myself happened quite quickly, but I realised that I couldn't afford to
rest on my laurels … I had a long, long way to go yet.

Wednesday 2 March:

My first thought for today: I think that being seriously fat could
be compared to having a mental health problem about twenty
years ago. People can see you have a problem, but nobody wants
to talk about it. It is a big, dirty secret.

My second thought for today: The way I see it, the food industry is based upon deception, and the same goes for the multi-million euro diet market. Why is there so much misleading information about the food we buy? For instance, certain ingredients have more than one name so half the time people don't realise exactly what they are buying and consuming. There are forty-two different names for the substance MSG alone, which I find incredible! Also, the weight values on a lot of food labels are not the exact weight of the product itself. There is an ingredient called Cellulose, which basically is wood pulp, and is used in bread and pastries to improve their texture, but you won't find it on a food label because it is not food. I am sure that this is barely touching the tip of the iceberg.

I was listening to Ray's show, this morning, and Paddy from **The Biggest Loser** was on it. They started talking about me. Now, that was weird, in a good way. My phone immediately started beeping with text messages.

Orla (my sister) is getting married in July, and I am beginning to think that I could be about twenty-eight stone for the wedding, which means losing another thirteen stone before then. It sounds like a tremendous amount, but based on the way things are going, I believe it is a fairly strong possibility. A second goal is to be eighteen stone for Christmas. From the reading at Motivation, I have around seventeen and a half stone of muscle, so I think I would look great at eighteen stone.

Actually, today I am really fired up. It occurred to me that it would really help my head to set goals. So, the above are my first two, regarding my weight. I am also thinking about two more, regarding exercise. For instance, there is a swimming race in Killaloe in September. Maybe I could give it a go? Plus I was thinking about asking Rob and Darren to do the Cork Marathon with me. You can do it in relays, and it would be great to do it with my brothers. I don't know, perhaps next year I could look at doing a full marathon?

I sent a copy of my diary, today, to Jenny Kelly, in Today FM, to give her a better understanding of what has been happening, but I'm not so sure it was such a good idea now. I used to be so closed off about this stuff, now I'm thinking about doing marathons and passing on my diary to be read by someone else. Yikes!

A woman wrote into the Ray D'Arcy Show, this morning, about having to go through IVF treatment, to get pregnant. She said that she was finding it difficult to be around other people and their babies. I couldn't help wondering if Shelly experiences something like this. It doesn't bother me though I do get mad when I see parents not looking after their children properly.

Thursday 3 March:

Okay, so I am going to fast forward where I want to be in twelve months time:

    Eighteen stone, and fit and healthy

    In college, or in a job that makes me happy

    Playing rugby for a season

    Competing in Strongman again

    And hopefully we will be blessed with children

    Obviously some of them are more important than others but

I do think the list is achievable ... well, except for the last one. Unfortunately I have no control over that.

I just had steak for lunch. Nowadays everything just tastes the same. It really sucks! I am dreading next Tuesday, Pancake Tuesday. I love pancakes!

What a shit day. I was so hungry I went to bed in an attempt to escape, through sleep, my pangs of hunger.

Friday 4 March:

I am starting to crack up. I'm serious. Everything I put in my mouth tastes like crap! Everywhere I go, all I see are petrol stations where I could buy rolls or muffins, and fast food places. And, for the life of me, I cannot understand it, but what I really, really want what I am utterly craving – is a bowl of Crunchy Nut Cornflakes. WTF! I rarely ate them before I started all this, so why in God's name are they all I want now?

I might eat my arm.

On the plus side I am bringing Nicole, my god-daughter, swimming tomorrow. So, that is something to look forward to.

This has been a horrendous two days. I can't take much more, I really can't.

Saturday 5 March:

It was a better day today, thank God! I weighed myself, 522.5lbs which means I am 1.5lbs off losing a grand total of four stone. The plan is to push hard at my training, here, at home, with the workout that I've devised myself, over the next few days so that I can break that by a few pounds. Then, roll on five hundred!

Monday 7 March: (Week 8, weight: 520.4lbs)

Total weight loss, so far, is fifty-seven pounds or 4.1 stone. I am so happy about hitting the four stone mark, and am considering whether to break out tomorrow to have some pancakes. However, I am waiting to hear from Jenny Kelly, about whether or not I'm on the radio next week. If I was I would really push the boat out to make it five stone by then, so I won't make a pancake-related decision until I talk to her. I mean, I'm not saying yes and I'm not saying no, although if I have a good day today I'd probably say no.

I have noticed that my flexibility has improved a good bit; I can reach further around my back. Unfortunately my knees are still pretty sore.

(Pancake)Tuesday 8 March:

I made my decision and it is final. I will have two pancakes tonight. I would rather make the decision properly and be happy about it, than breaking out at the last minute and feel crap with the guilt.

My energy is much improved today. I swam sixty lengths in the pool. Not bad at all!

When I came back home I didn't want to sit down, so I pottered around the house doings bits and pieces. This is good.

So, I have just had my two pancakes, and I have to admit I didn't enjoy them half as much as I expected to. I built them up in my head, how they were going to taste, and they fell short of my expectations. This is also good.

It took until early March before I started to feel the effects of the change in my diet. They say it takes your body thirty days to deal with positive or negative effects of your diet and it took me this amount of time before the sugar withdrawal symptoms eased and the benefit of my new healthy diet started to kick in.

Wednesday 9 March:

I was worried that I might feel guilty about those pancakes last night, but I don't. I made the decision, after a lot of deliberation, and it was the right one. Today I am glad to be back on the wagon again. Yee ha!

Swam another sixty lengths today.

Jenny rang to tell me I will be on the show next Wednesday. It was a bit of a weird call, mainly because I was in weird form and kept rambling on to her about nothing. Sometimes I have these brain farts.

My mate Deccy is running a charity boxing tournament and I'm thinking about signing up for it, as I've always wanted to learn how to box. I'm going to think about it.

Thursday 10 March:

Thanks to feeling a bit stiff and sore I did less than my usual sixty laps.

At 10am I went to Motivation to be weighed, which was grand since I am down another eight pounds, in weight, ten pounds in fat and up a pound in muscle. I am really happy with that.

It isn't urgent, yet, but I want to find out what to do with saggy skin.

Orla dropped Shelly's bridesmaid dress down to Mam's, she looked great in it.

Friday 11 March:

Well, I had a good and a bad session in the pool this morning. On one hand I did sixty-two lengths, breaking my record, and, on the other hand, this was this idiot of a woman who kept cutting into my lane and into the guy who was swimming alongside me. That kind of thing does my head in.

I think I might be addicted to Mario Bros on Nicole's DS.

This evening, on the radio I heard that there is a three-year waiting list for an appointment in the National Obesity Clinic. What a joke!

Monday 14 March: (Week 9, weight: 515lbs)

Okay, so in total I have lost sixty-two pounds/four stone six pounds

Nevertheless, I feel very heavy today. It's an odd feeling, like someone has slid ten pounds of weights on my back without telling me. I am sluggish and lethargic, which is not the best way to feel when I am on a strict diet and feeling positive is almost essential in preventing me from cracking and eating a rasher sandwich.

Tuesday 15 March:

Shelly and I are four years married today.

Despite having a good swim this morning, I am in a foul mood , but am doing my best to ignore it.

I went to Motivation and weighed in at thirty-six stone and ten pounds. This is three pounds down from last week, but my muscle mass was up and my fat was down seven pounds, so I was happy enough with that.

Siobhan, from Motivation, is coming with me to the radio studio tomorrow. Ray wants to talk to the both of us. I am going to try and get in a few extra workouts before then, but I still feel very heavy. Just my luck!

Wednesday 16 March:

Left home this morning at 6.15am, it was bloody freezing, and picked Siobhan up at the train station. We chatted the whole way to Dublin, though I think she was a little nervous about going on air.

When we got to the reception we were met by Jenny who asked me to bring the scales down to the studio. As usual everyone was really friendly and supportive. I weighed in at thirty-seven stone and a pound, which was a five pound difference from the Motivation scale, but I kind of expected that. The interview went really well, we had a great chat with Ray. After the show Jenny told me to put through my travel expenses for my last three appearances, which was unexpected, but much appreciated. She also mentioned about perhaps getting me a personal trainer.

Apart from enjoying the show I still was not in the best of form. Maybe because I missed out on my swim this morning I felt particularly heavy today.

Thursday 17 March:

Happy St Patrick's Day!

The sun is high in the sky and it is a beautiful morning. I felt
I needed to email Jenny in Today FM to tell her I was a little
worried about the personal trainer idea. What if it is someone I
couldn't get along with, or had little understanding about what I
am going through?

Friday 18 March:

Yeah! I hit a new personal record in the pool this morning, with
eighty lengths, and I felt I could have kept going but I was more
than happy with this.

I saw a funeral today and it reminded me of how much time
I used to spend thinking about dying, during those dark days,
imagining that my family and Shelly would have to get a super-
sized casket. I went as far as to worry about how nobody would
have been able to carry it which would surely have been doubly
distressing for everyone. The logistics of my funeral used to be one
of my biggest fears, but, thankfully, that is all in the past now. It
certainly is another bloody good reason to lose weight.

I was talking to a guy I know who told me that his brother is
going to train for the half-marathon thanks to my radio interview.
Somehow I inspired him to make the decision. I have to admit I
am really chuffed about this.

My legs are still giving me problems. I am starting to wonder if it has anything to do with the chlorine in the pool.

Monday 21 March: (Week 10, weight: 509lbs)

I have lost sixty-eight pounds to date!

Tuesday 22 March:

In Motivation, this morning, I weighed in at thirty-six stone one pound. Yep, I am pretty happy with that.

Spent some time, in the afternoon, reading back over this diary. So much has happened since I sent that email to the Ray D'Arcy Show. If someone had told me ten weeks ago that I would be down almost five stone and swimming every morning I would have called them crazy. A lot has certainly changed, just in the last couple of months, including how I feel about myself.

Wednesday 23 March:

I weighed myself, this morning, out of curiosity: 502lbs in my boxers; 509lbs in my clothes. This put me in great form and I swam eighty-four lengths of the pool, a personal best. I could have done more, but my legs were starting to cramp from being in the water so long.

These last few days, mood-wise, have been really good. It has to help that the weather has been gorgeous.

So, I have about three weeks, or so, before I start my boxing training. I want to work on my endurance, fitness and speed beforehand, so I am going to go online and find out how I can do this. I am also determined to be as light as possible, I reckon I could be under twenty-eight stone if I really got stuck in, which means upping my training to three daily sessions of thirty minutes, on top of the swimming.

Thursday 24 March:

Shit session in the pool as it was bloody freezing!

This afternoon I decided that I am going to do the 'Join Ray for 5k' run. Obviously I am going to have to walk it, which is something I am going to start doing immediately because I only have about two weeks to prepare for it. It is best for now if I keep this to myself, just easier that way. Also I cannot decide if I am going to do the one in Galway or Cork.

All in all I have set myself four goals for the coming months: the 5k in two weeks; starting boxing in three weeks; the Lough Derg swim (2km) in September; the Global Powerlifting World Championship in November, if I qualify during the summer. This is all, I feel, within my reach.

It was another great day. I did some gardening with Shelly, which is possibly a first, and then she went and burnt the ribs I brought back from the butchers. They tasted awful so we gave them to the dogs.

Hi Ho! Hi Ho! It's off to the gym I go!

Friday 25 March:

Day Sixty-eight in the Big Brother House! Seriously though, I do feel, sometimes, that I am living inside a bubble. Can I really be doing this for sixty-eight days now; it sure doesn't feel like that long.

The pool was busy this morning so I had to and sit in the sauna for ten minutes, to wait until it emptied out a bit. When I came home I followed up the swim with a quick fitness workout.

Damn you, Ray D'Arcy, I would sell my soul for a rasher sandwich, dripping with brown sauce.

Monday 28 March: (Week 11, weight: 507lbs)

Total weight loss is seventy pounds/five stone.

Ha! This morning I smashed my new personal record and swam a wonderful hundred lengths in the pool.

I was checking myself out in the mirror – another personal triumph, I'm not afraid of the mirror anymore – and I have to say that today was the first day I could see a physical difference in me, especially around the face.

It took me nearly five stone before I could see the difference in myself, so in the same way I didn't see it going on I didn't see it coming off either.

Tuesday 29 March:

I called over to see the lads, Deccy and Jeff, at the boxing club. They were taking some photographs to promote the place and they put me in to pose with Willie Casey, who is even smaller than Ray D'Arcy. Talk about Little and Large! Deccy is going to give me a few one-on-one classes, starting next Thursday. I am both looking forward to and dreading them. I mean I do not want to make an eejit out of myself, but, then again, fair fucks to me for giving it a go.

I am on a roll now. I spoke to a guy, Liam, who is involved with 'Cycle for Sick Children', telling him I was going to do it for them.

Friday 1 April:

Good old April Fools' Day!

I am still giving serious consideration to doing the 'Join Ray for 5k' event in Cork, next Tuesday. Am I in or out?

The 'Join Ray for 5k' run in Cork was a big milestone for me; it was something I would never ever have considered doing before I went on the *Ray D'Arcy Show*. Despite all the progress I'd made, doing something in public like this was still a huge step. I headed off early to Cork, and was fine in the car. In fact I was even excited about this, my first big event. However, once I reached the Páirc Uí Caoimh Stadium, my excitement went into a tailspin and I began to feel what can only be described as pure terror. Honestly, I don't think I've ever been as nervous about anything else, from getting married, to going on the radio that very first time.

Fortunately there were not too many people around yet, as it was only 11am, so I did my first lap quietly enough, thinking: *Okay, this is not so bad.* I had worried that I might not be able for the two laps. When I finished thirty-five minutes later I went to move the car. More and more people started to arrive and I got myself into another state. They were all slim and healthy looking and were, I'm sure, wondering who the hell I was. My heart was pumping like a steam train and I began to be afraid that I couldn't go on. Naturally I was the heaviest around and fretted that I looked like a fool. I thought I might even wait around until 2 or 3pm when most people would have finished and left for home. That's how bad it was.

The crowd of runners emptied out of the car-park and headed off merrily for the start line. They all looked like they knew one another. Talk about feeling lonely. I stood in the car-park, which was about four hundred metres away from the start and was doing my best to find some confidence. Just then, Shelly rang me and I remember saying to her, 'You just don't understand – I can't do it. Please don't ask me to do it!'

I was panicking at the thought of facing all those people. Standing in the car park I could clearly hear the PA from the start line; I heard Seán Óg Ó hAilpín, the hurler who was opening the race, tell everyone that it was not about the winning, it was about the taking part. Well, that was exactly why I was there; I just wanted to take part, to see if I could do it. His words, and the crowd's rousing reaction to them, inspired me to stay where I was. I was going to do this because I had to. So I walked out of the car park and up towards the start line; the race had started but that didn't bother me.

When I got going I was fine, although I have to admit I did stay on the path, out of everyone else's way. That way, if anybody saw me they would think I was just some guy out for a walk. I snuck passed the small crowd, at the start, and was going up the road when I heard some of the runners come around for their second lap. I kept to the side and kept my head down.

Ray D'Arcy lamped me straight away and came over to talk to me. This calmed me down, and I didn't mind at all when the more serious runners passed me by. Actually I think I may even have started to feel comfortable as I stuck to my own pace. After a while I saw that people weren't paying me a blind bit of notice, and the atmosphere was lively and friendly. Of course I had wondered if I might encounter any 'looks', but that wasn't the case at all.

I crossed over the finish line, with a bad stitch in my side and sore calves, but I finished!

As I made my way back to the car, in a daze, a girl came up and asked me if I was Gary from the radio. Her name was Paula and she was really supportive of what I was doing; we stood chatting for a bit. When we said goodbye I put the key in the car door, and that's when it suddenly hit me what I had just done. I had taken part in something that scared the life out of me, and involved being around lots of other people. Me, who, just a short while ago, had been too afraid to leave the house. I never would have believed I would be doing something like this by April.

After the race I spotted Will Hanafin and gave him a lift into town. Jenny Kelly had left a message of congratulations on my phone so I rang her back to tell her how it went.

On the drive home I had plenty of time to think about my performance and I did feel a bit of a twit that I just didn't plonk myself in the middle of the crowd as a proper participant. But, still, I did it.

Wednesday 6 April:

Oh, am I sore today, but I went swimming which helped.

Everything hurts, from my bum down to the blisters on my feet.

Nevertheless, I am strongly considering going to Dublin, to do the Join Ray for 5k run on Friday. The way I see it, I had to do the Cork run just to see if I could. Now I want to take part in a run where I forget about myself and be free from worrying what other people are thinking of me.

Ha! I was on the internet, reading about the things that can happen when a person loses a lot of weight. Men's penis-size increase by an inch, for every stone they lose. Well, if that's true I'll be hung like a donkey this time next year. We'll wait and see.

After a bit of soul-searching, I decided to build on my experience in Cork and do the Dublin 5k. I was disappointed in myself for not starting with everybody and I was determined to do it properly, so that Friday I headed off to Dublin about 8.30am. I had to email Jenny about taking part, because the race was full. I arrived at Irishtown Stadium about 11am and told the guy on the gate that I was with Today FM, which allowed me to put the car in the car-park.

It is nice to be able to write that I was not as self-conscious as I was in Cork. I took a quick walk around both to check out the route and loosen up my muscles. A couple of others were doing the same thing and recognised me. They wished me well though I couldn't help thinking that they didn't really know what to be saying to me. But that was okay.

I hung around the car park until ten minutes before it was due to start, I headed to the track where I found my nervousness waiting for me. There were a lot of runners and all of them tiny in comparison to me. I kept my head down and reminded myself that it was all about being there and taking part. There was a bit of a moment when some smart-arse kid yelled out, '814 to win!' That was my number. Instead of folding up in embarrassment, I thought, *Fuck you! I have already won just by turning up.* Only God knows how many demons I have had to fight, to reach this stage. And the truth of it was that I felt happy, and did not experience one jot of shame about standing in the crowd of superior competitors.

As soon as the race got underway I was alone once more, everyone taking off at a great pace. I nearly got lost, more than once, but I found my way again. It was different from Cork because of my familiarity with this part of Dublin. I knew exactly how far I had come and how long I had left. When I got back to the stadium I was swept up in a cloud of support by a group of twenty people or more who came and walked the last lap with me. It was like a Hollywood ending to my run. I was so moved that as I approached the finish line I broke into a jog, which my body did not thank me for. In any case I finished it in under an hour and was suitably chuffed about that. Job done!

I got home about 6.30pm and spent the evening chilling out, feeling that I more than deserved to.

Sunday 10 April:

Had a crap day yesterday. My legs were pretty sore and I had a blister on top of a blister, but I managed to go swimming with Shelly and Nicole. Then I dropped Shelly to work, came home and felt so bad that I had to go to bed for a few hours. I was curled up into a frozen ball and I don't think there was one part of my body that did not hurt.

When I managed to get out of bed, I took pain killers and went over to watch the match with Dad. Still feeling crap, I came home and rested until it was time to collect Shelly from work. This is when I really started to feel ill. We got home and I was shaking with a fever and feeling so, so weak. Shelly rang Mam, who came over immediately, but I don't remember her being there. They said I was talking all sorts of rubbish, with the fever. Shelly rang the doctor who advised her to call an ambulance. Fortunately I came around after a bit, took Paracetamol and began to feel a little better.

I still felt pretty sore and weak when I work up this morning so I went to the doctor who gave me antibiotics for a bad tonsil infection. He told me to come off the diet for five days, but I had tea and toast last night **and** today. That is enough, as far as I am concerned.

Monday 11 April: (Week 13; weight 496lbs)

In spite of still feeling under the weather I went and swam. Today, on top of everything else, I have a mouth ulcer and a cold sore. Ugh!

I watched last Friday night's **Late Late Show** on the RTE player. There was a guy from Motivation, in Wexford, who had lost 'nearly twenty-five stone'. This annoyed me. What he had actually lost was twenty-three stone and I just wondered why he couldn't just use that figure instead. It is a fantastic result and he should be thrilled with that, instead of putting a sort of negative spin on it, by calling it something that it isn't: it is two stone off twenty-five stone and nothing to feel bad about.

Tuesday 12 April:

I went to Motivation this morning and discovered I was two pounds up on last week. In short, I was gutted but Helen, the franchise owner, told me it was because of the antibiotics.

It has been thirteen weeks since I made a list of the stuff I wanted to do. I am going to update it now. So, here is what I want to do;

Charity boxing fight

5km Shannon/Lough Derg Swim in September

10km, and then a half marathon, and then a full one

Take part in the Powerlifting World Championship in Limerick, in November

Bodybuilding show

Tough Guy Race, held in the UK, in January 2013, which is the hardest race in the world.

It is probably a mad list of goals but I have now done two 5km runs so I can only build on that. I have to start somewhere!

Wednesday 13 April:

Apart from a cold sore and mouth ulcer I am feeling pretty good. When I picked Shelly up from college she was in a strange mood, and I spent ages trying to find out what was wrong with her. Finally she admitted that one of her friends had just found out they are pregnant with twins.

We talked about it some more this evening. She was in tears. All her friends are having or have had babies and still none for us. I kept telling her that our time would come while inside I was praying that I was right. This is one of the reasons I am doing this, to become healthy so we can have children. I honestly don't know what I'd do if, after losing all the weight, we still couldn't get pregnant. Actually, I can't even think about that scenario.

Monday 18 April: (Week 14; weight 491 lbs)

I am down eighty-six pounds, or six stone two pounds.

Boxing starts tonight, and I have more than a few butterflies at the thought of it. I think there is going to be about thirty of us altogether.

Oh ho! I am just back from boxing. It was the hardest workout I have ever done, and coach said he was actually starting us off easy this week. The sweat rolling off me could have filled a bucket. Nevertheless, I managed to do everything, even the running.

By this stage, I was beginning to feel really relaxed about my visits to the Today FM studios. I really appreciated the amount of support Ray and the team lavished on me. I was finding that the interviews gave me an opportunity to talk openly about the mistakes I'd made as well as assessing how far I had come, and thinking about my future. The listeners provided a huge, faceless network of reassurance and encouragement. In the past I had only ever received this from my wife and family and was humbled now to be recipient of so many good wishes from virtual strangers. All those people who texted, rang in or wrote on my Facebook page, they can never know how important they became to me. Meanwhile the monthly weigh-in was something to focus on when the days sometimes turned into something of a battlefield where I had to try and find a way to distract myself from

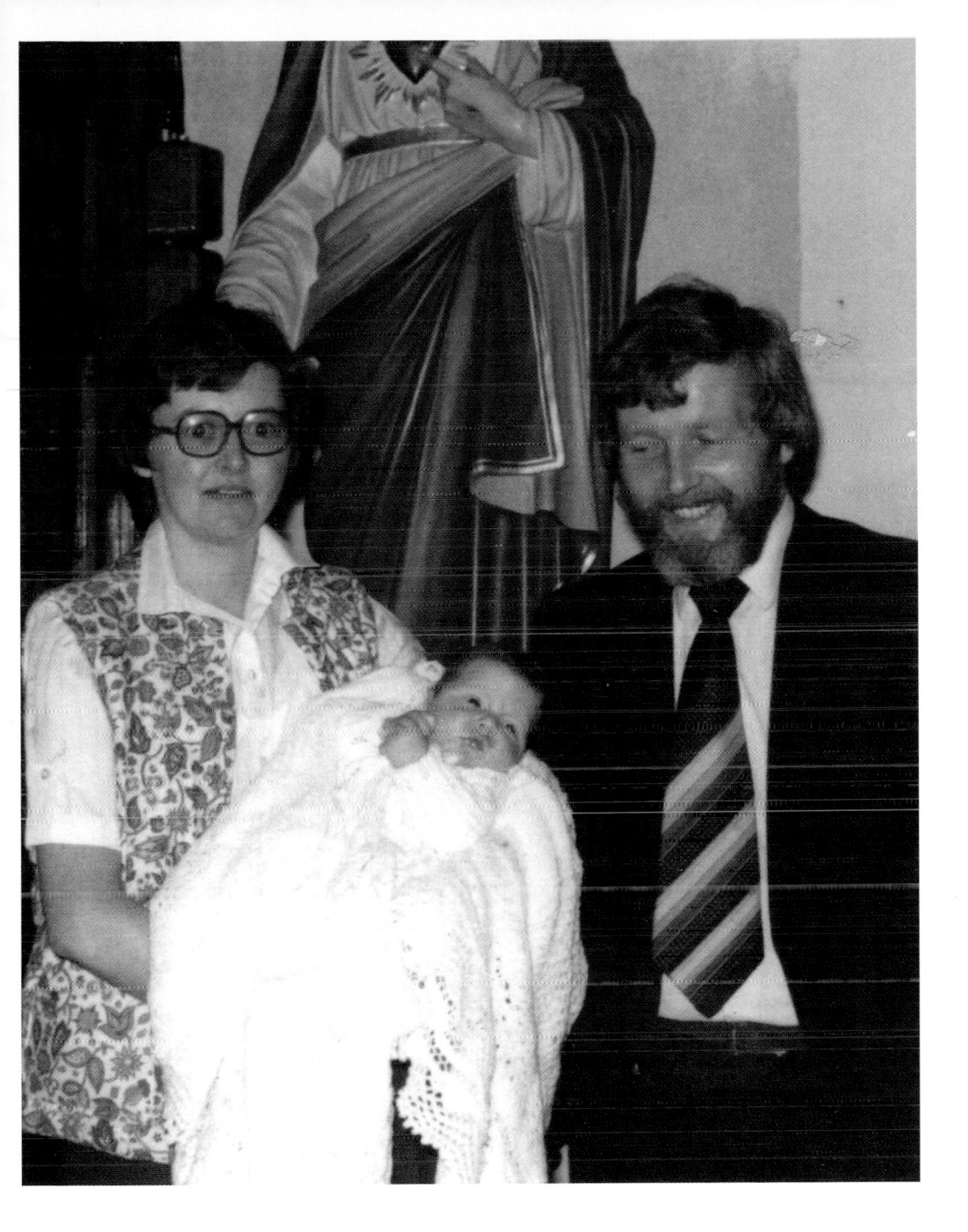

Above: Me at my Christening in St Marys Church, Limerick, with my Mam and Dad, Lucia and Peter.

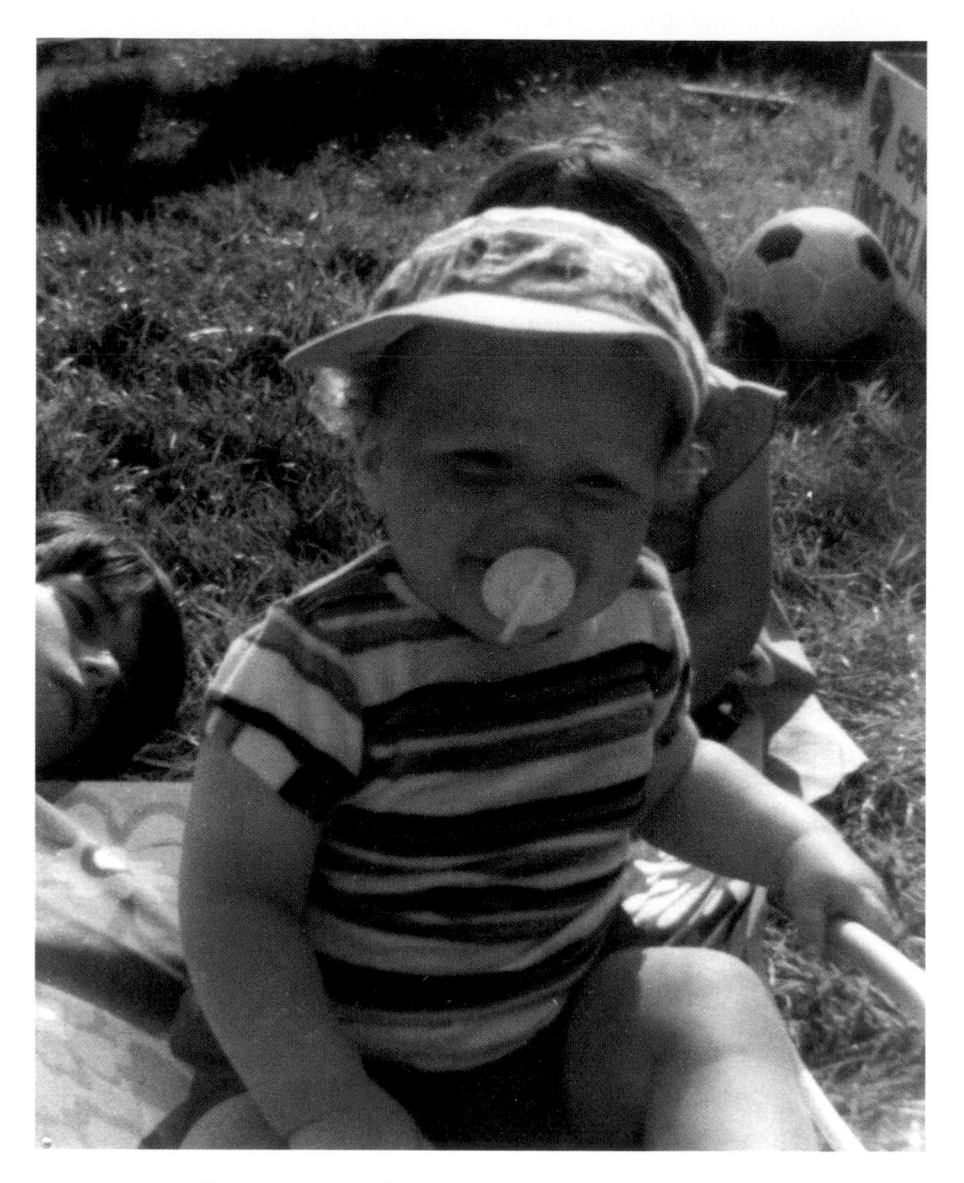

Above: Playing in our garden as a two-year-old. I had a very happy childhood.

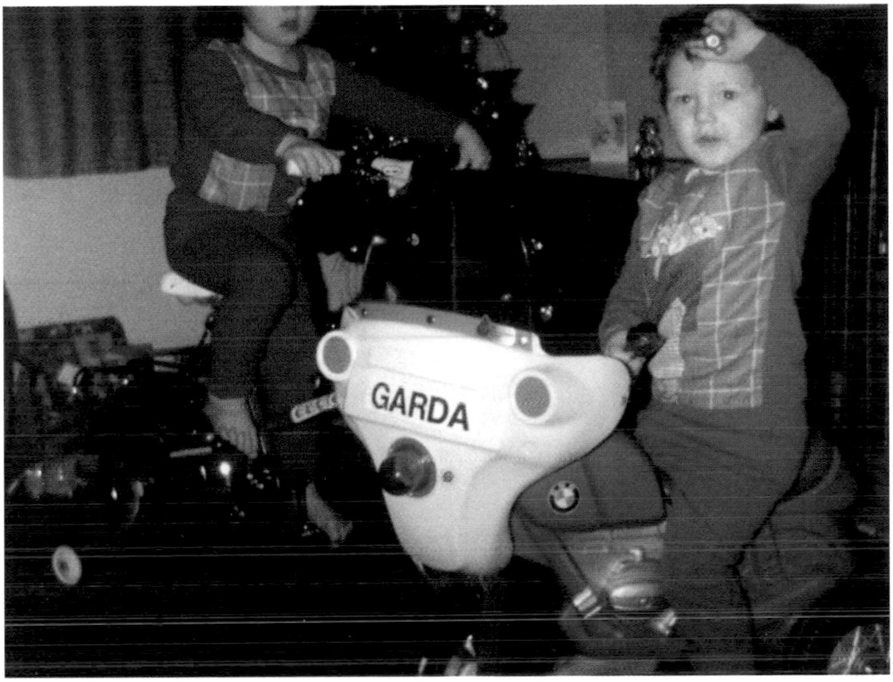

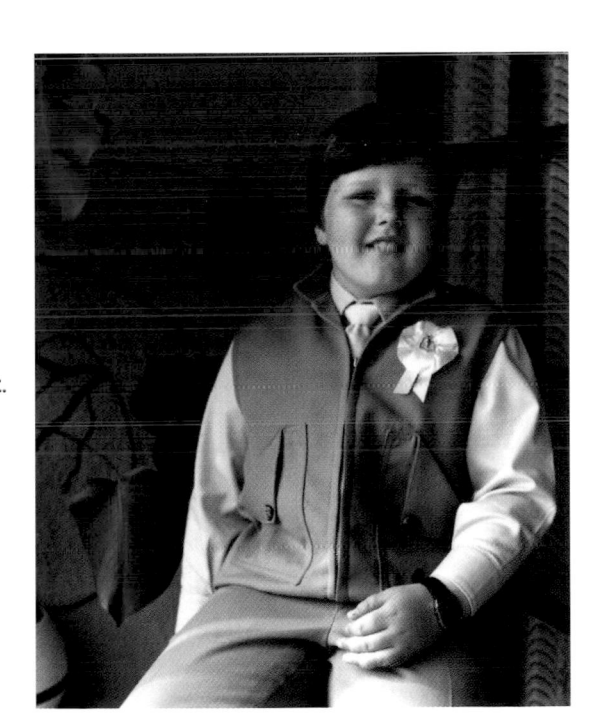

Above: Aged four. Christmas morning with my sister, Orla.

Right: At my Communion in my custom-made green suit. Though I was too heavy to buy a Communion suit off-the-peg, at this stage I wasn't really conscious of my weight.

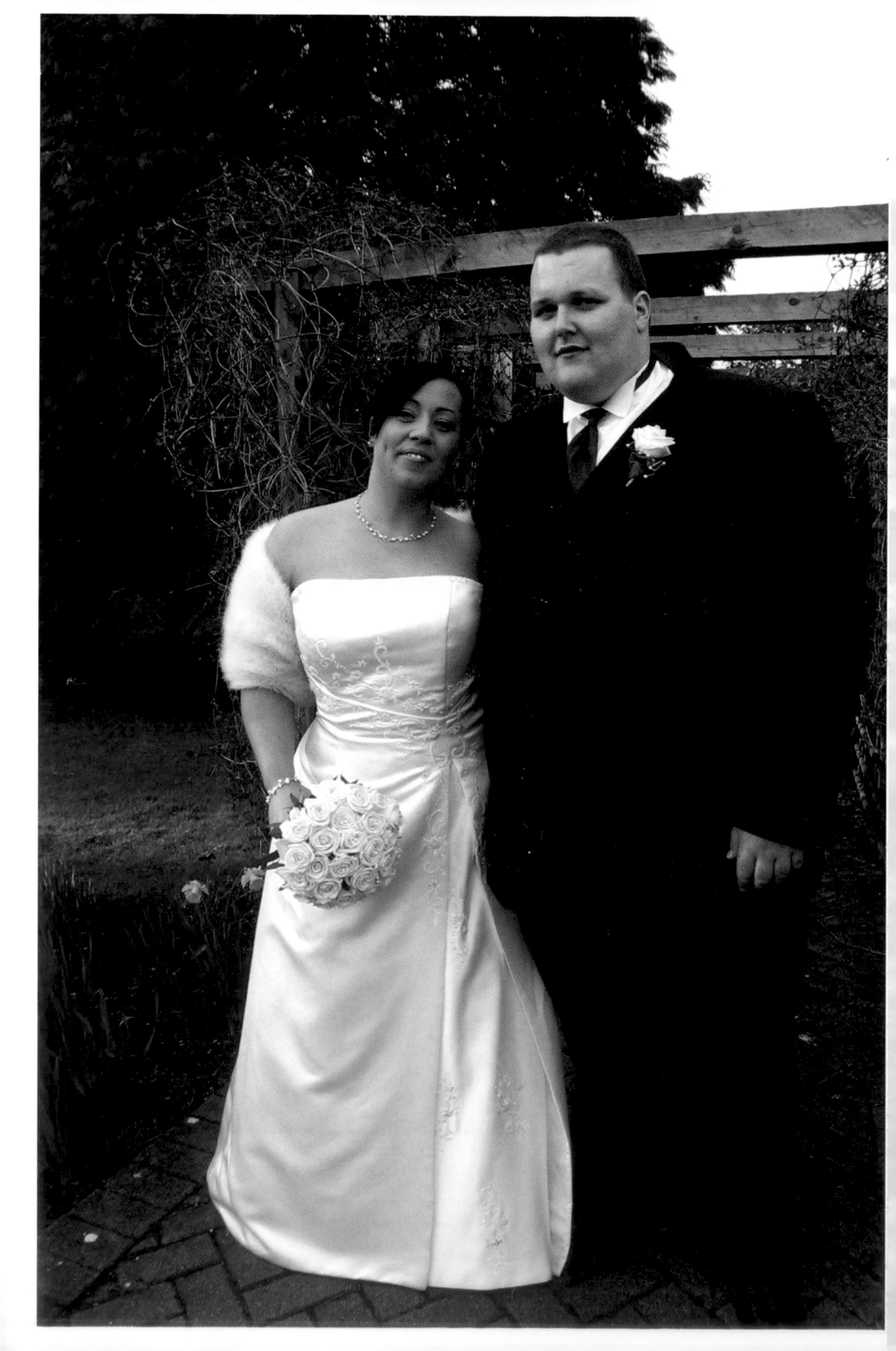

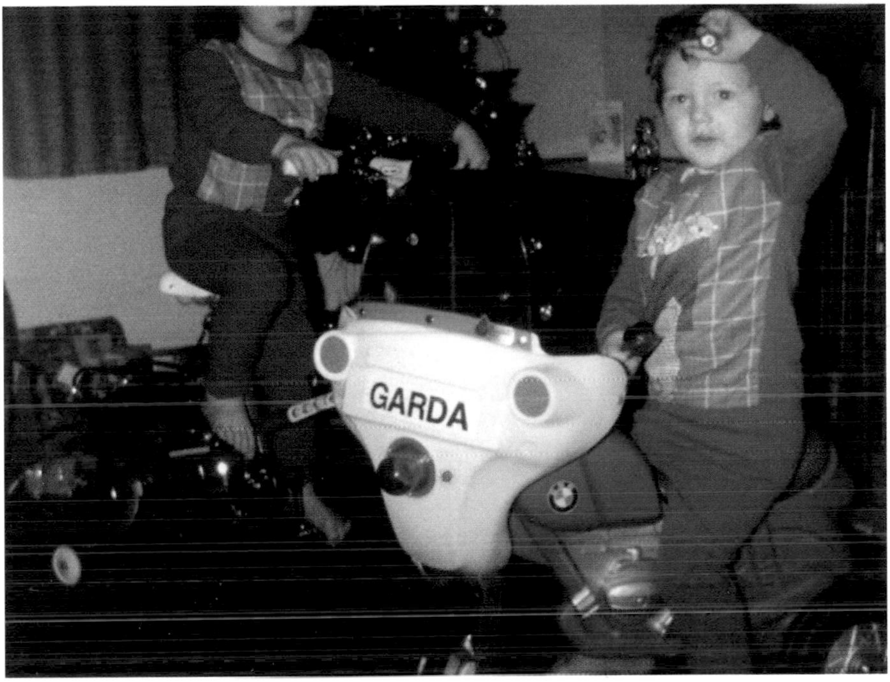

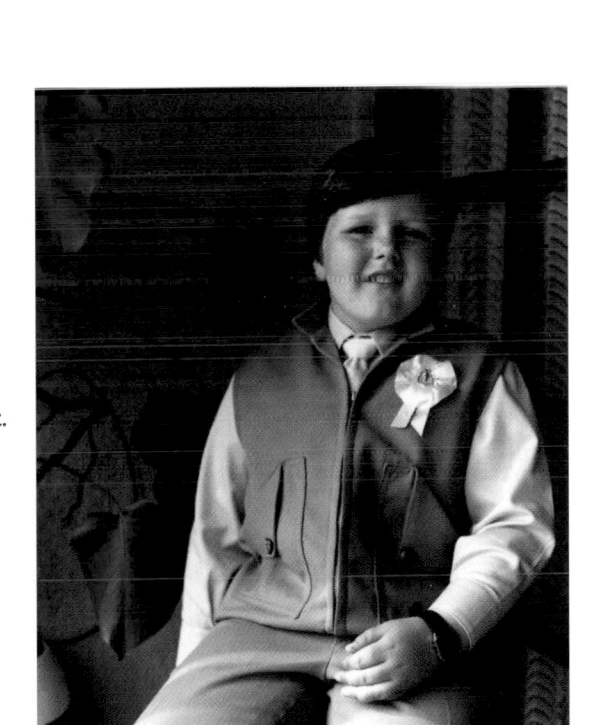

Above: Aged four. Christmas morning with my sister, Orla.

Right: At my Communion in my custom-made green suit. Though I was too heavy to buy a Communion suit off-the-peg, at this stage I wasn't really conscious of my weight.

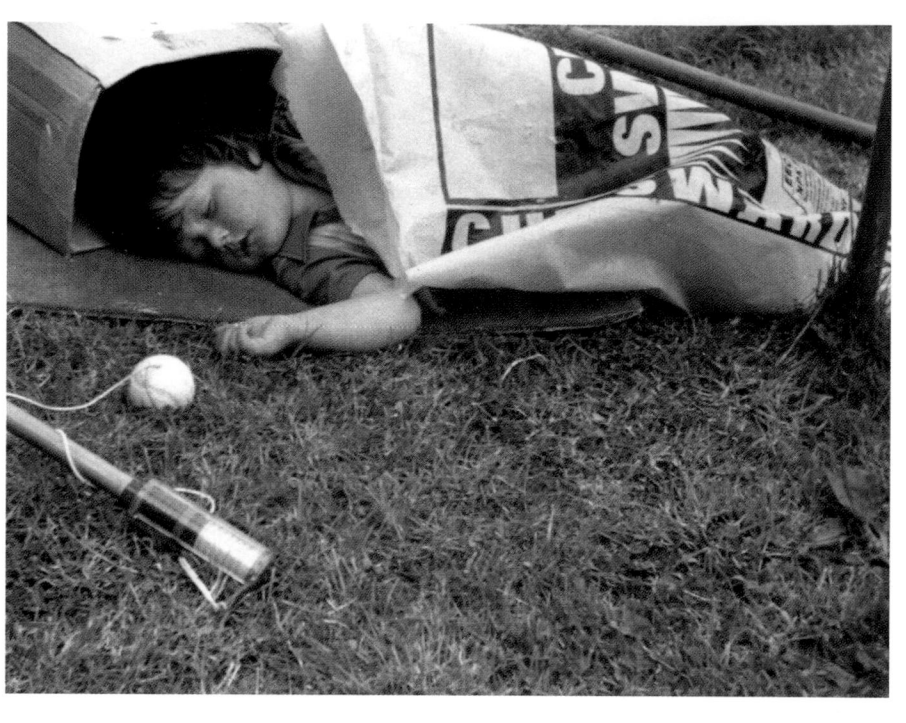

Above: Aged seven, worn out from playing!

Right: Aged twelve. My first year in secondary school.

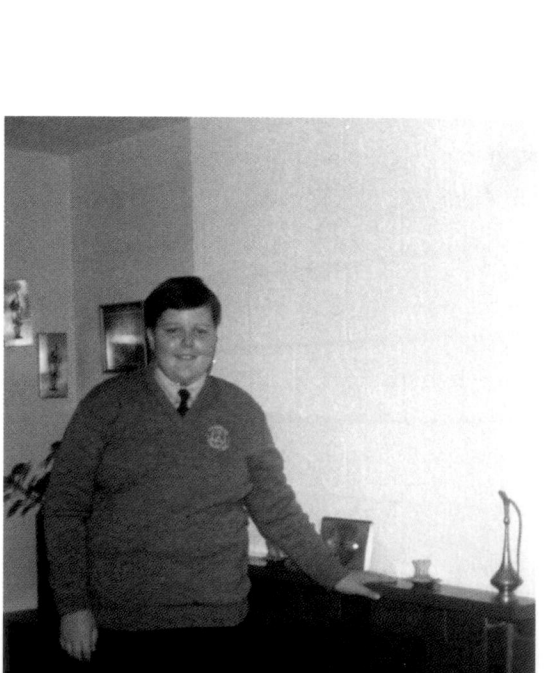

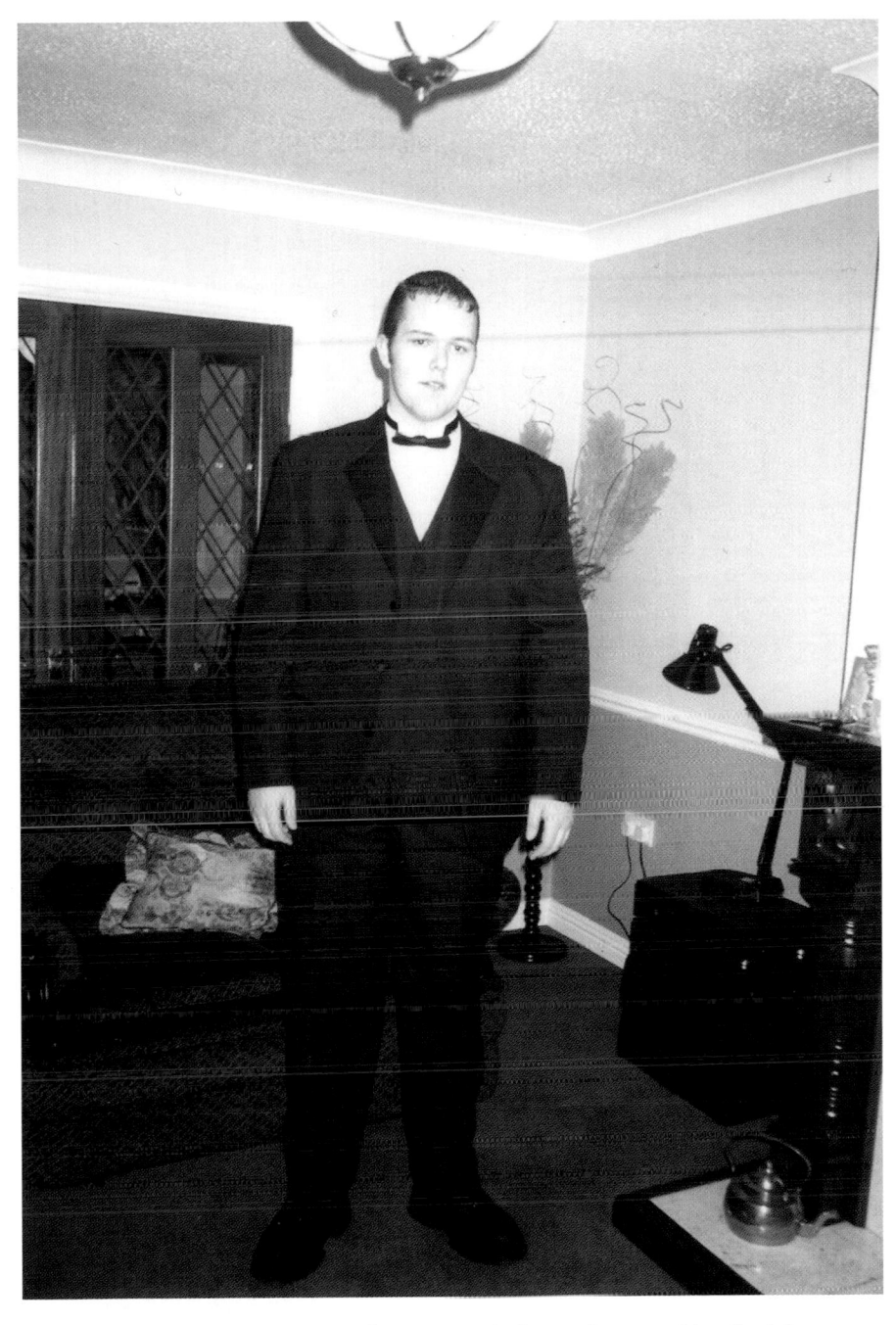

Above: Aged nineteen, after my crash diet, going to a friend's debs.

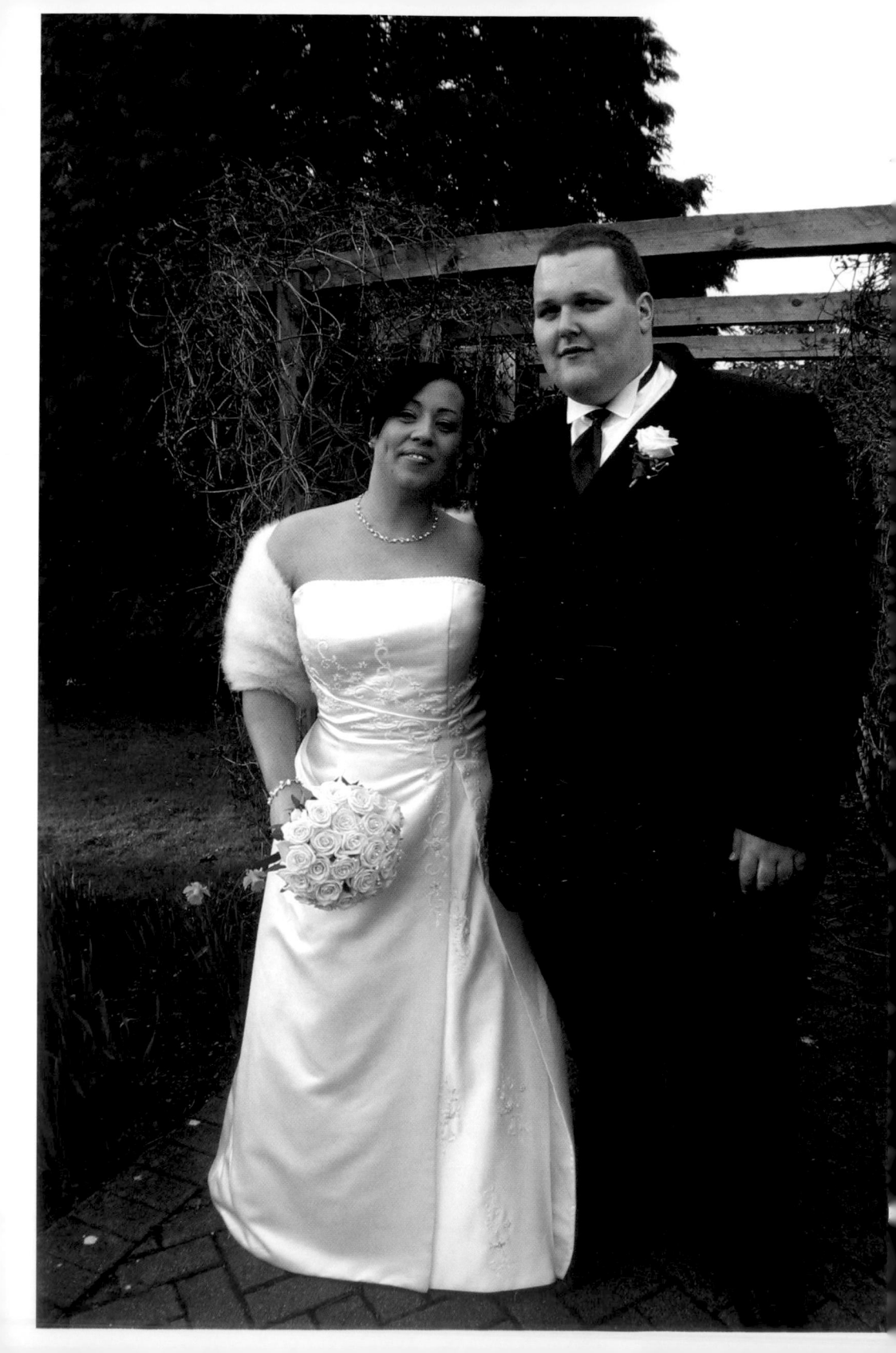

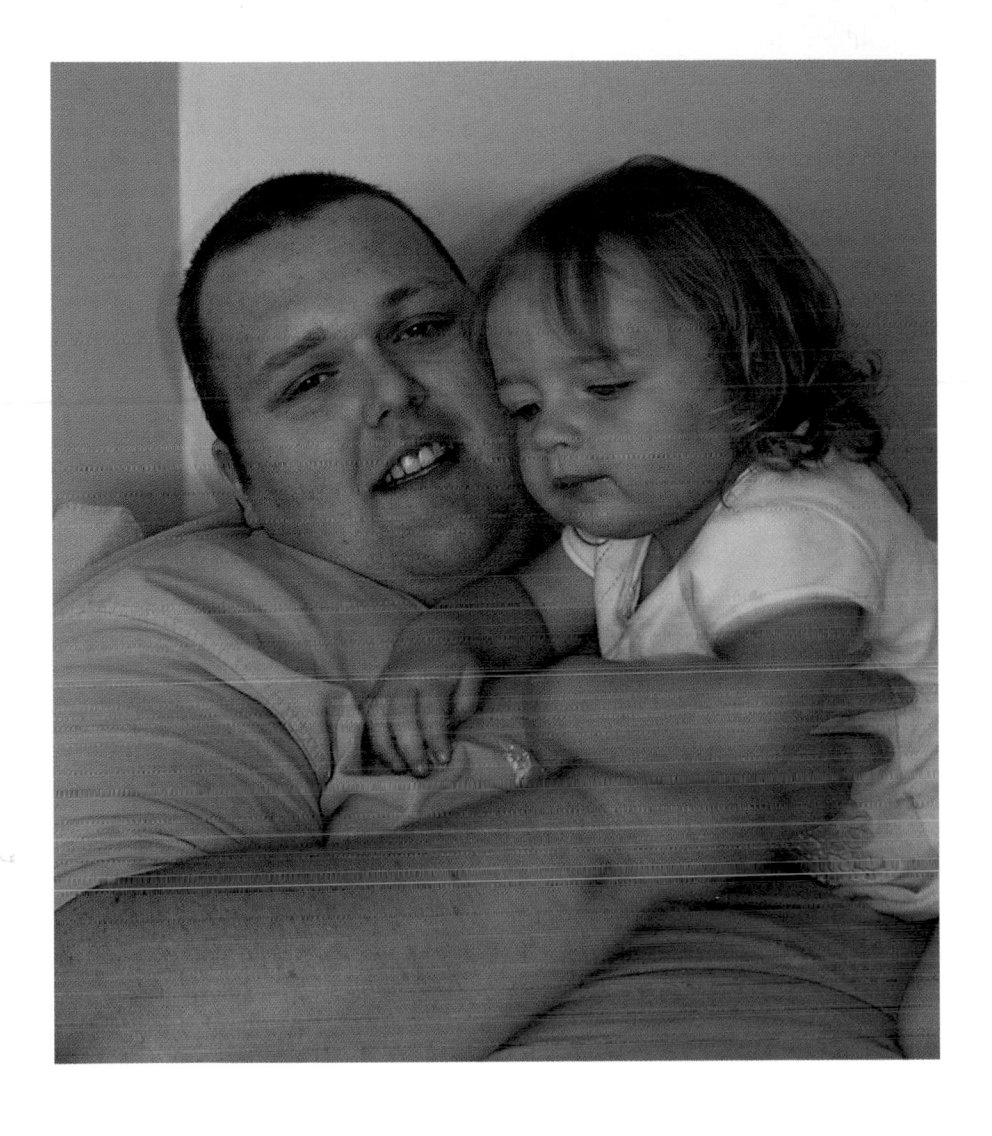

Above: with my niece and god-daughter, Nicole. I was very heavy at this stage, and quite depressed, but Nicole could always cheer me up.
Left: my wedding day, with my beautiful wife, Shelly.

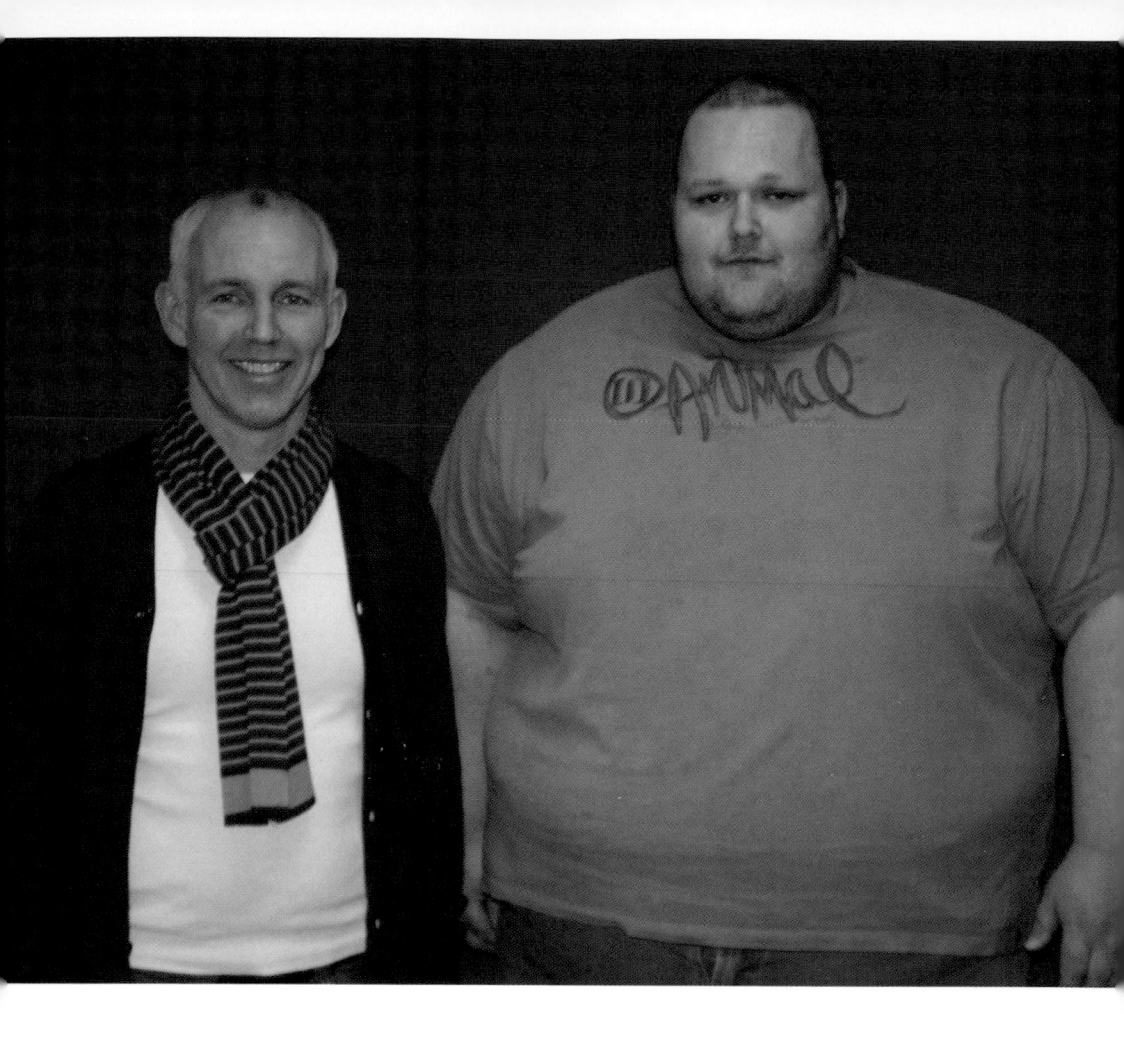

Above: With Ray D'Arcy at the beginning of my journey on 17 January 2011; little did I know where it would lead. Ray and his team have been such a support to me.

how hard it was. The thought of being weighed on-air and everyone hearing how much weight I had lost since the previous month proved to be an excellent incentive for me.

Thursday 21 April:

I went swimming and then later on I went and did a private boxing session. It was hard though there was no running involved. My muscles ached after only a couple of minutes.

Newsflash: This is a very special day indeed. It is the first time, in a long time, that Shelly can get her arms all the way around me. The fact that she couldn't was one of those things that I would not allow myself to dwell on. But, now she can!

Friday 22 April:

After a great swim, this morning, I took Nicole to Smiths Toy Store, to buy her a present instead of an Easter egg. She is so funny with the stories she comes out with.

This evening I ate two hot cross buns! I decided that I am going to take three days off the diet as I am struggling a bit with the fact that the sugar in the coating of the antibiotics is messing with my weight loss. To be honest, I feel more than a little fed up today, and it must be because of that.

Rob (my brother) introduced me to his new girlfriend, Becky. I am sure he was in a sweat in case I said anything, but I was very well-behaved. I will wait a bit before I start slagging them. Ha!

Saturday 23 April:

Went swimming with Nicole and Shelly, then I dropped Shelly
to work and brought Nicole back to the house. She spotted the
weighing scales in the car and asked me why they were there,
and I explained about being on the radio show. She went quiet for
a second and then asked, 'Are they nice to you?' I looked at her,
puzzled, 'Who?' and she replied, 'The people on the radio'. 'Oh, yes',
I nodded, 'They are very nice to me'. 'Do they throw flowers at your
feet?' I was a bit gobsmacked at this question but it turned out
that she was watching a Tom and Jerry cartoon, where they were
on a stage, doing a play, and when they left, the audience threw
flowers at their feet. It made me laugh.

    I had a nice evening with Shelly; we had homemade burgers for
dinner, followed by cider. I had three cans and feel quite drunk,
after months of abstinence. It was too sweet and very gassy,
which made me feel sick.

Sunday 24 April (Easter Sunday):

Today was my first Easter Sunday ever without eggs, and I did not
ever care because I knew Mam was cooking me a turkey dinner.
And a lovely dinner it was, turkey, stuffing, roast potatoes and
vegetables. I ate it really slowly, savouring every mouthful and
then stopped when I felt full. In other words I only ate half a plate
of it. It gave me a good feeling to know that I could trust myself
like this.

Monday 25 April (Bank Holiday):

What a boring day, but at least I had boxing in the evening. I am back to normal, on the diet, from today, after finishing the course of antibiotics last night. Although my tonsils still feel sore and swollen.

Tuesday 26 April:

I was weighed in Motivation today, and am up by a pound, which is not bad considering I came off the diet.

Shelly and I are going to see Peter Kay (British comedian), at the O2, on Thursday. I am a little concerned about being in a big crowd and having to squeeze into a seat.

My throat is really sore; I think I better go back to the doctor's.

Wednesday 27 April:

There is another race I want to do. It's the Turf Guy Race, and involves a 10k track split into a 5k run and a 5k obstacle course. I would have to go to Mayo to do it, but it's not on until November which gives me a few months to prepare for it. Maybe I will ask one of the brothers to do it with me.

I had another great boxing session tonight, tough but highly enjoyable.

Thursday 28 April:

I went to the doctor today about my tonsils and ended up telling him about us trying to have a baby. He said that he had never heard of excess weight causing fertility problems; however our last doctor had said the fertility issues were because of my weight. I don't like to think about what else could be wrong.

We are just home from the Peter Kay show. The seating wasn't too bad, though I still felt quite self-conscious in the crowd, and dreaded anybody having to make their way pass me in my seat.

Friday 29 April:

Sometimes I wonder where I am going with all of this, or where it will finish, if it has to finish. Obviously I have my desired weight as my goal, but losing weight alone is only half the point, as my other reason was to improve our chances of conception. Okay, so that may not happen, which is something I can't think about for long, because the idea of Shelly and I being unable to have children is a terrifying one. In the meantime, however, it did occur to me that I would love to use my experience to show other people that it is never too late to lose weight and get fit.

Around this time, Today FM sent me the details of some people who contacted them wanting to talk to me about what they were going through. At first I was in two minds about it. I liked to think I could reach out to other people, after all I had been through, but I couldn't stop worrying about whether or not I could be of help. It was a big responsibility. In the end, I decided to do my best, and I got in touch with two guys who had given their contact details to Today FM. I rang one of them and emailed the other. When I was giving my story so far, it gave me a new appreciation of all that I had achieved. Maybe it is impossible to help someone without helping yourself at the same time.

This is the email I sent; it was the first time that I felt I had something real to offer another person.

Dear XX

That is great news that you joined with Motivation, the books and tapes do help.

The good thing is that you don't really go hungry, it can just get a bit repetitive but you won't mind that once the weight starts to drop off.

The other thing I would say is to listen to your consultant, and no one else. Everyone has an opinion on the subject of losing weight, and while their hearts may be in the right place, you will hear a lot of well-meant nonsense.

You wanted to know about my swimming. Well, I suppose, because I went public, going to the pool was not a huge issue for me. Without a doubt, you will be stared at, but you probably get that anyway, so does it really make much of a difference? You are doing this for you, so fuck what others think. You will be surprised at the support you receive from the most unexpected places. It does help to have someone to go with you, for the first few times, for moral support.

Yes, I would tell people what you are doing. As I say, you will receive plenty of support, which is brilliant, but also know that there will be the jealous begrudgers too. That is all I can say about that!

The other thing I would suggest is to keep a diary. I also take a picture of myself, every two weeks, though, to be honest, I haven't actually looked at my photos, I don't want to see them, at this point.

You won't really notice the weight coming off, so just be prepared for that. I have lost six stone and I still don't see much of a difference. On the other hand I notice little things, for instance, when I was driving my belly used to touch the steering wheel, now there is about gap of a few inches. It is those stupid little things that make me smile.

Also, make a list of the rings you would like to do once you have lost the weight. Why wait until next year to start your list. It doesn't have to be a marathon, just something like a 5k walk, that's what I did.

Break down your total desired weight loss into milestones: the first stone, the third stone, and then one hundred pounds It helps to make it a little less daunting.

There will be days when you feel great and then the down days, but just push through them. Sometimes I feel like a lunatic but you have to keep going forward.

After fourteen weeks my life has improved in so many ways. It is crazy how much can happen in a short amount of time. Look at it this way, by Christmas you could well have lost twenty stone, and just think how different your life will be.

I really hope this has been of help to you. Keep in touch.

Gary

Monday 2 May: (Week 16, down six stone and 12lbs)

Woke up late this morning, so I skipped swimming because I knew the pool would be crammed with children.

Tuesday 3 May:

I am seriously down today, I have to just bloody snap out of it.

Wednesday 4 May:

I swam and then did a great boxing session, where I did ten by sixty metres runs. I feel much better today, the only way I can describe it is that I feel in the zone, and utterly motivated. Not sure what yesterday was all about.

Friday 6 May:

After a savage boxing session, last night, I feel very sore today. The thing is, no matter how hard the boxing is, and how sore I feel on waking up, mentally I am wide awake, alert and ready to go.

I went to the pool but I wasn't able for much, though I did feel a lot better for going along.

Big News of the Day: I weighed myself and am down a hundred pounds!! I am over the moon and feel like shouting it out from the roof of the house. All those times when I thought I might not get to this point and now I have. I was so excited I emailed Ray D'Arcy.

There were more media requests, from the **Limerick Leader** and TV3, who want to do a follow-up on me.

Saturday 7 May:

I got up at 3.30am to do the 'Darkness into Light' 5k, here in Limerick. It was sad to see so many people who have lost a loved one to suicide. The atmosphere was quite emotional.

I didn't manage to run any of it but I did meet Rob, from boxing, and kept to his pace which was a bit of a push for me. However, I beat my Dublin time by ten minutes, finishing in forty-eight minutes, so I was happy with that.

When I got home I found a blister on each foot. I went back to bed and up at 9am to go boxing. It was a hard session, both my legs and my arm were giving me difficulty, but I pushed through it so it made a great start to the weekend.

While I have been in 'the zone' for the last while, after the walk and boxing this morning, all I can think about is food. Shelly is off to do her last exam for college, and then she goes to Cork for Orla's hen's night. In other words I am home alone tonight and do not want to be in this mind frame.

Thank goodness! I was saved by watching **The Biggest Loser USA**. Watching other people go through this is inspiring.

Monday 9 May: (Week 17, weight; 476lbs)

I am down 10 lbs, which is a great boost to my confidence. This should be a good week since I am now definitely off the antibiotics, and hopefully that will be it with them. That situation was head-wrecking, to say the least.

When I went to the pool they told me that my membership is up. This fucks me up since I just don't have the money to renew it.

Tuesday 10 May:

No swimming for me this morning. I don't know what I am going to do. By the time the bills are paid there is very little left.

Motivation weighed me today. I am down 102lbs so I am happy with that.

Dr Donal O'Shea was on the Ray D'Arcy Show this morning, talking about weight loss; he and Ray mentioned me which gave me a kick. I always get a buzz when I hear Ray talking about me, he sounds like he is genuinely proud of me. The doctor said that if a person weighs forty-one stone and takes the route of a gastric bypass, they can only go down to twenty-eight stone. I am so happy I am doing this the old-fashioned, hard way. Plus, the benefits of doing it this way involve having the time to address the stuff that was ruining my life. Nowadays, I am much less self-conscious, I am fitter, happier, and don't suffer from the frequent bouts of depression that plagued me throughout the last couple of years. I am now able to look at the photos that I took of myself, at the beginning of this year; it is still not an easy thing to do, but at least I can do it now.

Shelly and I went to the bank today to try and sort out the mortgage. I feel like we are being given the run around, from pillar to post. It is so frustrating to feel so out of control regarding these things.

Tonight I started to think going back to college. I'm going to have a look at what's on offer at the Limerick College of Further Education and the Limerick Institute of Technology. This was on my list of things-to-do. I see Shelly really enjoying her course and feel inspired by her. College could provide a chance for a new career, or, at the very least, give me a bit of a choice for the future while keeping me busy during the recession.

<u>Wednesday 11 May:</u>

Because I had to sign on this morning, I had to miss swimming, which wasn't the most pleasant start to the day. Afterwards I went to the dentist for a check-up. He delivered the awful news that I need a few fillings that are going to cost me €290.

Well, I am just home from a disappointing session at the club.

For weeks, now, I have been dodging a female partner, but my time ran out and I was paired up with a girl called Siobhan. Call me old-fashioned, but I couldn't hit her, so I was just tipping her. While I tipped her, she wasn't so accommodating and was quite happy to hit me! I just couldn't get over the fact of hitting a woman — probably a good thing!

Then I sparred with one of the guys and he gave me a few good boxes. I managed to get in one or two and I learned a lot from him during our brief session. There was a two-minute break before I sparred with one of the faster boxers, whereupon I fell apart after he knocked me in the eye, actually touching my eyeball. It was excruciating. Next he caught me with a low blow. I was absolutely raging, but instead of channelling the anger into good boxing, I just clammed up.

This has been a nightmare day, from beginning to end!

Friday 13 May:

Killer cramps in my legs and groin woke me up at 3am.

Despite the fact I can't really afford it I knew I would have to go see a physiotherapist. Luckily enough I managed to get an appointment for 11am this morning. He gave me acupuncture and deep-tissue massage, which is quite painful during it but leaves you feeling stoned and perfectly relaxed afterwards. Then, I had a wonderful surprise. When it came to paying he wouldn't take any money from me because I gave him a mention on the radio, the last time I was on. Happy, Happy Days!

When I got home I emailed Jenny, at Today FM, about getting

me a personal trainer. When it was first mentioned to me I was a bit sceptical but now I think it could be really helpful. I want to suggest this guy that is taking part in the charity boxing, Chris Delooze from TriFit gym. He has a great reputation and seems like a really decent bloke. Plus he is also a swimming coach, so I think he would be perfect for me.

I collected Shelly from work at 6pm and we called into see Nicole, in my parents' house. They were having dinner: steak, carrots and roast potatoes. It looked and smelt bloody divine!

Damn! I have just realised that the queen is in Dublin next week. In other words finding a parking space is going to be a nightmare.

Saturday 14 May:

Shelly had to work early so I called down to Mam's and took Nicole out to the park. She brought her football. God, it was so great to be able to run around with her and not be tired.

After I dropped her home, I was on my own for the rest of the day so had a lot of time to think about stuff. I still cannot understand how I did not see how shit my life was. I also thought about Shelly and what I put her through with my dark moods. How has she stayed with me? One of the wonderful consequences of this new regime of diet and exercise is that it has really changed our relationship for the better. Because I am losing weight I am happier and healthier, and my confidence had improved too, resulting in the atmosphere at home, and between us, being a lot lighter. I decided that I should only look forward now, with Shelly, and leave the crap and regrets firmly in the past.

We chilled out tonight in front of the television, to watch the **Eurovision Song Contest**. Poor old Jedward were robbed.

Monday 16 May: (Week 18, weight; 465.8lbs/33 stone and 2lbs)

So I am down eight stone, though I know that when I am at Today FM, on Wednesday, it will say I am only down seven and a half stone, because I will be wearing clothes. It has been a slow month thanks to the antibiotics. The main thing now is to push hard for Orla's wedding on 1 July, which gives me six weeks to get down by another three stone. That will be bloody brilliant. To think that back in January I would have settled for losing four or five stone by now. You never know what you can do until you start doing it.

Wednesday 18 May:

I got into the car at 4.50am to drive to Dublin and found that I had plenty of room in the seat belt which made me beam widely at that hour. Fortunately traffic was quiet and I was on Digges Lane by 7am. With two hours to spare I went for a walk to loosen up my legs.

It is funny how normal it has become, me going into see Ray and the team. Today's show was particularly special. Sometimes I cannot believe how supportive they all are. I start to feel like an eejit because I don't know how to handle all the nice stuff they say to me. The simple truth is I cannot overestimate how important they have been to me.

When I got home I listened back to the show and was again touched by Ray's manner toward me, including when I had gone, he was still talking about how well I was doing. I felt so good I whipped out those photos of myself to study them properly and, for the first time, I do see a difference in my body size.

Thursday 19 May:

I went back to the doctor who put me on stronger antibiotics. He wants me to cut back on some of my supplements as he thinks I might be having an allergic reaction to one of the ingredients.

This evening I listened to yesterday's Ray D'Arcy Show again, after hearing Ray talk about me this morning. It is just nuts that I have someone like that who believes in me one hundred per cent.

Friday 20 May:

This morning I received a cheque in the post from Today FM for my travel expenses, so I am going to use it to renew my membership at JJB, which means I can start swimming again. Happy Days!

Saturday 21 May:

A good day! I signed up for nine months with the gym and thoroughly enjoyed my swim this morning. I don't think I even realised how much I missed it.

Monday 23 May: (Week 19, weight; 33 stone and 6lbs)

The antibiotics are seriously pissing me off. I am up four pounds.

Where is the justice in the fact that when I was forty-one stone I was never sick, but now that I have lost eight stone there is constantly something wrong with me. Fuck! Fuck! Fuck!

I went swimming again this morning, so good to get back into my routine. In the evening I went to the boxing club and had a hard but great session. I also spoke to Chris; he is going to start working with me from next Monday. We'll train together two or three times a week.

Tuesday 24 May:

This morning I drove to Killaloe, for the launch of the i3 Open Water Swim, at Lough Derg, because I wanted to learn more about it. As it was finishing up a lady approached me. She was a big lady who knew all about me, and asked how I was getting on and what exactly I was doing. We were having a grand chat when this guy came up and congratulated me on my achievements. Before I could thank him, he turned to the woman, whom he knew, and said, 'Well, you might get the lead out and do something about yourself now'. I was absolutely gobsmacked. The poor woman looked shocked, and very near tears, while I tried to think of something to say but, in all honesty, I was too taken aback to respond. Why on earth do some people think these sorts of statements are helpful to anyone?

Wednesday 25 May:

Shelly came swimming with me this morning. In the car, afterwards, on the drive home, we were listening, as usual, to

Ray's show. He mentioned me in relation to a problem one of the listeners had contacted the team about. It was a young girl, a teenager, who weighed twenty-two stone. There was talk about her eating habits being enabled by her family, which annoyed me. My weight is my fault, and no one else's. I honestly don't believe that obese people are big thanks to their families. Perhaps it is a relevant point when it comes to overweight children but apart from that I disagree with it being used as a reason. Regarding this particular girl, her mother died two years ago and she probably feels very lost and lonely. Plus her family no doubt think that she is going through enough as it is, so they won't want to hassle her further about her weight. That's my tuppence worth on the 'enabling' issue. Really, I have always hated that word!

I look back at my life and think nobody 'enabled' me to eat. I made my own decisions and I have to take responsibility for that, I hid how it was affecting me very well from those who loved me most and I was pretty good at it too

Thursday 26 May:

Ray mentioned me again on the show. It is surreal to hear them talk about me; I always feel that it is somebody else he is praising.

Shelly went to her bank this morning to find her social welfare payments had been stopped, with no word of notice. How do they expect people to survive like this?

We had a good evening though. We went to a table quiz that was raising funds for Pieta House. Rob, from boxing, was running it. Out of a total of fifteen teams, we came in third last but there was no shame. Everyone else had four people on their teams while there was only the two of us.

Friday 27 May:

Five weeks to Orla's wedding! I'm starting to get excited about it; it should be a great day.

Mam and Dad are thinking of bringing Nicole over to England, for a few days, while Orla and James (Nicole's parents) are on honeymoon. Shelly and I might go along too. I would love a few days away and it is the only holiday that we are likely to get. Also, since we are staying with family, it shouldn't affect my diet too much.

Though I had lost more weight in the past four months than I would have believed possible, I had decided that just losing weight wasn't enough, I also wanted to be fit and healthy. So in June, I found myself walking into the TriFit Gym, for my first session with someone who was to become a huge part of my life, trainer Chris Delooze.

From the beginning Today FM had wanted me to work with a personal trainer, but I was a little reluctant after watching the trainers on weight loss TV programmes. I did not want someone who would shout at and berate me, and was unsure if I could find a trainer who genuinely wanted to work hard with me. I first met Chris at Limerick Charity Boxing, he trained Jeff, one of the boxing coaches who I know and have a lot of time for. Because Jeff always spoke about Chris in glowing terms I knew he had to be good. But then, everyone speaks well about Chris. He's the sort of guy that women love and men would love to be. A good-looking Aussie, he's absolutely easy-going, charming and is an accomplished sportsman. I decided to ask him would he take me on. However, deciding to ask and actually asking are two different things. For two weeks straight I meant to approach him but always bottled out of it. Finally, one day, before training I asked him. He seemed not to know much, if anything, about Today FM, merely saying that yes, he would love to work with me.

He put me to work immediately, making me wear a heart monitor, to assess where I was physically. The monitor was a comfort to me as there was the worry that I might push myself, or be pushed, too much beyond the realms of safety for someone my size. I could do neither a single press up nor sit up so I was starting at the very beginning. Those first weeks, and months, were unbelievably tough and it was here that Chris performed his miracle, pumping me up with self-belief that I could do anything I wanted to. I had the determination, to be sure, but I needed someone who could make me see what I could do. He is so genuine in his attitude, and hugely encouraging, which is essential in a situation like this, that I found myself trusting him completely. Some days he would jump onto an exercise bike beside me to chinwag about how things were going for me. Recently he told me that his approach was primarily to always get me to finish each session, not allowing me space to give up. If I had been allowed to give up on one session, it would have made it so much easier to give up on another session. Instead Chris was determined, via 'tough love', if you like, to build up my confidence. So, if I finished one session, it made it that much easier to finish the next one.

As I began to improve, which took time, I found I could do a sit up.

A little while later I found I could do several, and so it continued on like that. Before I knew it I could do several push ups. These seemingly minor accomplishments were big victories for me. Don't get me wrong, Chris is a very tough trainer, his sessions last between sixty and seventy minutes, in which you are kept moving non-stop. But he was right. When I managed to finish these sessions, I would experience a surge of disbelief and then pride in myself.

Monday 30 May: (Week 20, weight 32 stone and 11lbs)

Twenty weeks! Where has the time gone? And what a great start to this week, I am down nine pounds from last week.

I went swimming at 9am and it was good because I'm starting to pick up my old pace from before. After that I had my first session with Chris, at TriFit. I have to get a heart rate monitor so he needed all my details: weight, height, age. He also asked me what my desired weight was and what level of fitness was I looking for. Because it was our first session, it was sort of a 'test day' to assess how I was. How I was, was shattered! Halfway through I felt light-headed. His session reminded of the tough workouts on **The Biggest Loser.** On the other hand, it was absolutely exhilarating.

When it was over I went home and straight to bed, rested for a couple of hours, before going out again, this time, to boxing. My legs are like jelly tonight.

Tuesday, 31 May:

The pool was quite busy this morning, which ruins my fun. Shelly came with me and we both experienced frustration when people kept cutting into our lanes. As it emptied out, it was like a scene from the film **Cocoon**, as we were definitely the youngest in the pool then, by about thirty years or so.

I am stiff and sore this morning but I feel fresh and alive. Physical training is just great for the head. I think it helps to keep me positive about myself, all that adrenalin or whatever. I used that word 'exhilarating' about Chris' session yesterday and that is exactly how I feel today. When I think of the hours I put in, sitting on the couch, watching television for hours. How could anyone be truly happy from just doing that?

Shelly has lost a stone and a half, and it really shows.

Wednesday 1 June:

Swimming, personal training and boxing today, and I was still sore from Monday.

This morning Shelly saw her doctor about what our next step should be in regards to having children. He is going to refer us to a fertility clinic in Cork. Because we can't afford to go private, and pay, we have to apply to them and hope to be selected for treatment. God, I hope this is going to work. It does seem to be the case that I am the problem here, but why? Weight or no weight, the doctor said, there must still be something wrong, so we also need to go and see a specialist. No matter what it turns out to be, I would much rather know than just be worrying about all kinds of possibilities. I have heard so many different theories by now and am fed up with it.

Shelly emailed the Cork fertility clinic (CFC) tonight.

Thursday, 2 June:

For the next three days, I am helping out with the EPC Powerlifting Championships, in Kilmurry. It was tough, long day today but it was lovely to bump into people that I wouldn't see too often, since I only meet them in relation to the powerlifting. They all came up and congratulated me on what I was doing.

The fertility clinic rang Shelly this morning, after receiving her email. A nurse talked her through the process and is sending out all the forms today. We need to have our blood taken so that it can be analysed at the lab in UCC (University College Cork), and once we have done all that they will give us an appointment to come in. Fingers crossed that they can give us some answers!

Saturday, 4 June:

Thank God this was the last day of the Championships because I am exhausted and ache all over.

My weight has fluctuated like mad this week. I wonder if it is due to an increase in muscle from the increase in training. It certainly cannot be my diet since that has been going perfectly. Also I have sweated buckets, over the last three days, at the Championships, and I would have expected that to result in the loss of a couple of pounds or so. I was 454lbs on Thursday and 460lbs today. Now, that is harsh.

Sunday, 5 June:

I would not normally swim on a Sunday morning as the pool
is always jam-packed with children but I was desperate since I
had not managed to get to the pool in a couple of days so I took
a chance. It was the right decision! I beat two personal records: I
did thirty-two laps with the front crawl and swam an impressive
grand total of 116 laps.

We have Nicole coming tonight for a sleep over.

Monday, 6 June: (Week 21, 32stone and 8lbs)

So, I am down three pounds and I suppose I should be happy with
that, but I'm not. I just can't figure out if the fluctuating weight is
down to an increase in muscle or stress.

Nicole came swimming with Shelly and me, which was great
fun and a nice way to relax.

I spent the afternoon doing some jobs around the house.
They had needed doing for ages but I was too heavy and unfit to
even think about them before now. It was just simple stuff, like
cleaning out presses in the kitchen and front room. I even got up
on a ladder and changed a few light bulbs, fairly rejoicing in my
newfound freedom. These were the kind of things that I had not
been physically able to do in over two years. Shelly had always
done everything, and I mean everything, from the ordinary stuff,
cooking, washing, polishing, hovering, and changing light bulbs,
to the bigger stuff like plastering. Therefore, I could feel only
positive and pleased with this particular achievement. Plus, I was
neither sweating like a pig nor out of breath.

My brain has been in overdrive since last week. I wish I could take a break from worrying over things that I have no control off, like, for instance, whether we can have a baby, whether I can pay off my debts, what does the future hold me employment-wise, and so on. Honestly, it is driving me mad!

<u>Tuesday, 7 June:</u>

I took it a bit easier in the pool, this morning, since I was working out with Chris, weighing in with Motivation and boxing in the evening. A full day indeed!

A package arrived from the fertility clinic, this morning, to do with taking our bloods. It is up to us to get it to UCC.

At Motivation, I weighed in at 454lbs, which involved being down nine pounds of fat and up four pounds of muscle. This, at least, explains the ever-changing scales' figures over the last few days, so I was happy enough with that. Siobhan took a height measurement, I'm 6ft 2inches. At my heaviest I probably would have been a little shorter than that because the joints would have been compressed beneath the weight.

Chris gave me a tough work-out in the afternoon, with six sets of four exercises, for the upper and lower body, all involving much movement. It was hell! I had to go straight to bed when I got home.

TV3 rang me about going on their show next week. I told them to contact Jenny because it is the same day that I'm up with Today FM.

As I'm sitting here typing this, I feel now that I am in two minds over the weight result today. It is great that I am losing fat and increasing muscle mass but I don't know, I hadn't really expected this. What I am getting at is, this can only lead to a dramatic change in appearance, with less fat and a lot more muscle. It should look well, all right, but I sort of feel that it caught me off guard.

Shelly went down to Mam's tonight, for a fitting in her bridesmaid's dress. She looked amazing!

Right, I'm tired. I need to go to bed now.

Wednesday, 8 June:

God, I ache all over today. The pool helped a little, but not much.

Boxing went well tonight, my fitness is definitely improving. Yeah!

We booked our flights to England today. I'm looking forward to it, a deserved holiday with Shelly, my parents and Nicole. The last time I went on holiday I didn't want to leave the hotel room because of my size. Wow! So much has changed since then.

Thursday, 9 June:

It was a good swim, this morning, my pace was fast enough and I felt really good after it.

In the afternoon I had a storming session with Chris. I'm starting to feel that I'm getting the hang of it now. Feeling very pleased with myself in this regard.

I had to go to the bank where one of the girls on the desk told me that I had inspired her to join Motivation. I wished her the very best with it.

Okay, so here is how it is. I need to cop on. For the last few days I am been obsessing about my weight. For once, and for all, I need to believe that last week's result – with the loss of nine pounds of fat and the increase of four pounds of muscle – was a good one. I have to concentrate on not worrying constantly about the figure on the scales and, instead, focus on the plain fact that I am getting increasingly fitter and healthier. The niggling voice in my head keeps reminding me that I won't make the loss of ten stone for the next Ray D'Arcy Show nor will I hit thirty stone for Orla's wedding. However, I have to understand that I am doing my best and snap out of this doom and gloom. I do not want to be fixated on the scales or I will lose my sense of perspective about this, about what is important and what isn't. It is probably easier to write that down as opposed to actually doing it but it is simply another important thing that I have to work on.

Thanks to my head-wrecking mood I am in two minds about whether I want to do the TV3 show or now. It hasn't been confirmed yet, at any rate.

We're doing the bloods test for the fertility clinic Friday week and then I have to drop them immediately out to UCC.

Friday, 10 June:

My brain is still wrecking my head. I went shopping today and a woman, who I vaguely recognised, came up to me. It turns out she was in my class at Art College and that was a long time ago. Anyway she started asking me about the diet and told me that she and the girls in her office are all following my story. Honestly,

I really don't know what to say at times like this. I know I should just accept this sort of conversation as a positive thing, which it surely is, but today all I felt was embarrassment at the fact that she knew I had let myself get to over forty-one stone before I finally did something about my life. Is this a normal reaction? It just happens sometimes, that when a person is being friendly and supportive, all I feel is shame at how bad I allowed things to get.

Roll on for happier thoughts tomorrow!

Sunday, 12 June:

I took a day off from exercise. We went up to Mam's for dinner where I had beef, broccoli and cauliflower and watched everyone else enjoying that along with roast potatoes and gravy.

I am feeling pretty disgusted tonight due to the fact that I found an area of skin, under my arms, that has now become loose and baggy. It looks bloody awful, I feel sick just sitting here writing about it. There must be something I can do about it. I swear to God, I do not want my body to look like that, I would rather stay fat. Honest!

Monday, 13 June: (Week 22, weight; 448lbs)

I am down eight pounds from last week, which makes a total of nine stone three pounds.

FED UP.COM!

I know I should be delighted with hitting the nine stone mark, but I feel like I can't catch a fucking break. When I lose weight I get sick. Plus I have the most disgusting skin in the world. Where is the justice? I just want to stay in bed and pull the blankets over my head.

Boxing helped clear my head a little. Shelly has gone home to Tipperary for a few days so I'm home alone.

Wednesday, 15 June:

The alarm went off at 4am but I had been wide awake for about a half hour before that. I got up, had a shower and got into the car for the drive to Today FM. As usual I was there a whole hour early, I just hate the Dublin traffic so I will do anything to avoid it.

I was even earlier the last time and just spent the time sitting in the car, watching the staff arrive for work. At one stage, over the last few weeks, Ray came out to get himself a coffee. I was sure he spotted me but I didn't salute him so he probably didn't realise it was me. I have this worry that they might think I'm some sort of stalker and will cross boundaries of familiarity. Or am I being stupid? I'm half-laughing as I write this. I mean, are they business or personal acquaintances? I don't know. Is this an Irish thing, or is it just me over-thinking it?

Anyway I went in at 9am, bringing my supplements to give them an idea what I eat. TV3 sent a camera man and presenter to take footage of me in the studio. The show was really good, the more I do it the more I enjoy it. Once again I was blown away by the amount of support I received. We spoke a lot about feelings today, which is ironic after the last few days I've had. To be fair, I do think that this is where the biggest transformation is taking place, for me at the moment. People think that I am being very hard on myself, when I give out about not losing enough weight in a week and so forth, but I can't help thinking that it is a good thing to be honest enough to point out my failings on air. I think it helps me to deal better with them, so there is a positive outcome.

I made it back home in time to watch myself on TV3. I hope the audience has a better understanding of the training I am doing.

Friday, 17 June:

Shelly and I went swimming this morning and, on the drive home, we were listening, as usual, to Ray D'Arcy, who mentioned that there was an article about me in **The Sun** newspaper. Ray referred to me as 'Our Gary' and then corrected himself, saying that it sounded patronising. However, I like it because it makes me feel that I am more than just a story, plus, I think it is fair to say that we do have a bit of a bond at this stage. Anyway, God knows that I have been called much, much worse than that.

We had a meeting with MABS (Money Advice and Budgeting Service) so I am not in the best of mood as I sit here. It was a thoroughly depressing experience, having to listen to where we stand financially. Basically, our financial situation could be summed up in one word, 'Fucked'!

I have been thinking about the past, like when I first noticed I was fat and when I first went on a diet. I going to write out a timeline of things, not sure why, but it might provide some sort of exorcism of negativity.

Tonight I went and tried on some old clothes and it turns out that I will have a CHOICE of stuff to wear for Orla's wedding. Yippee! This is a big moment. My wardrobe is far from spectacular but to have a choice of old clothes, that I haven't been able to wear in ages, is as good as being able to go out and buy new stuff. So, I will be wearing a white shirt, dark trousers, tie and maybe my suit jacket. I will see how it sits on me nearer the day.

Monday, 20 June: (Week 24)

Shelly and I got our bloods done and drove to Cork this morning. We chatted on the way down and back about having children and it proved to be an emotional day, which was unexpected since all we were doing was dropping our bloods in. I suppose it is the thought that we have taken the first step on what could prove to be a long journey, with no guaranteed happy ending.

It was great to get out and box tonight, as it helped to clear my head.

Wednesday, 22 June:

If I had any idea how this day was going to go, I would have stayed in bed.

I was wide awake at 7am so I got up and went swimming.

Shelly had to go out for a while so I took the opportunity to try and write down some stuff from my childhood. I couldn't believe the amount of memories that flooded back once I got down to it. It was upsetting to remember back to the day in third year when I accidentally showed off my belly to the class and that teacher, who laughed and laughed.

Fortunately I got to work out some of my upset during boxing, though I did get my ass handed to me by Kevin, my sparring partner, since my head was in such a mess.

On the way home I decided to call in on the parents, just for a quick visit. I wanted to ask Mam about dates, to see that I had remembered them correctly, and I also wanted to be sure that I had the right reason why I ended up seeing the dietician in Limerick hospital. Then, before I knew it, I found myself opening up properly to Mam and Dad, telling them about the dark stuff that I had done my best to hide from them, like the looks of the disgust and the constant name-calling when I worked as a bouncer. We talked for hours and while it was a release, or relief, to tell them about the bad times, it was also bloody painful to see the shock and concern on their faces, apart from anything else.

I presume that I'm undergoing some sort of process, all this delving into my past and opening up to my parents, of all people. However I couldn't describe it as being a pleasant one. It makes sense, though; if you push bad feelings deep down inside you there surely has to come a day when they make their way back to the top, allowing you to release them. I mean, how else are you to get rid of them?

Thursday, 23 June:

If I thought yesterday was difficult, it was nothing compared to today.

When I woke up this morning, Kerry (one of our two dogs) was going mental outside. I went out to see what was wrong and discovered that Becky did not seem able to come out of her kennel. I told Shelly that if there was no improvement by the time I got back from swimming I would bring her to the vet.

Well, she looked even worse on my return, so I dropped Shelly into work and brought Becky over to the vet's surgery. My heart sank when the vet reckoned it was cancer, and it was in the late stage, as in too late to do anything. She told me to bring her to the bigger clinic, in Raheen, for tests to confirm the diagnosis. After I brought Becky in I rang Shelly, telling her that the dog was just dehydrated, she was on a drip and they were doing tests. Rightly or wrongly, I could not tell her the truth, not when she was at work.

I went boxing at lunch-time and when I was finished there were a load of missed calls on my phone, some from a landline and some from Shelly. I rang her first and she was in a terrible state. When the vet couldn't reach me he rang her and told her that Becky had leukaemia and it was terminal. Needless to say, Shelly was devastated, which I think I found more distressing than anything else. I felt so useless.

At 3.45 I met Chris for a work-out; it helped me forget about Becky for a short while.

I collected Shelly from work at 5.30pm and we went straight to the vet, to hear the most horrible news that Becky needed to be put asleep right away. We were shocked though understood it was the best, as neither of us were prepared to allow her to suffer any longer.

They gave us some forms to fill out, which I did because I didn't want Shelly to feel like she was responsible for having Becky put down. We were allowed some time alone with her, to say our goodbye. She was already lifeless, like she had already left us. Our beautiful, bouncing lab retriever went to sleep at 7pm on Thursday, 23 June, after giving us a fantastic eight and a half years.

It broke my heart to see the state Shelly was in. We called into Mam's on the way home, and everyone was very gentle and kind to her. When we finally got home Kerry knew. She sniffed around for Becky and, after a few minutes, went and curled up in a ball on Becky's lead.

Friday, 24 June:

Shelly is absolutely in bits. All I want to do is make everything better and I just can't. I collected Becky's body from the vets and drove to meet Shelly's mam in Nenagh. They are burying her at home beside Pebbles, Shelly's old dog. Poor Nicole was also devastated when she heard the news. I think it is good for someone her age to understand a bit about death. She insisted that Mam bring her up to see Kerry because she was worried about her being all alone.

Ireland AM rang me this evening asking me if I would be available to go on their show on Monday morning but I said no. I can't think about stuff like that after yesterday and today.

Saturday, 25 June:

I don't know if it is to do with what has happened but I sort of feel that I have hit some kind of brick wall. I am struggling even to type these words, for the lack of energy and interest. If I had to describe how I feel right now, it would be something along these lines: unmotivated, shit, and overwhelmed. It all just feels too much. I want to just go to bed and pull the blankets over my head.

Shelly had to work today but she's off tomorrow and I'm determined to do whatever I can to make her happy.

Sunday, 26 June:

I went to the boxing club for the first Sunday session. One of the best things about boxing is that it is a great way of getting rid of anger. It was a great work-out, although I am still, mentally, feeling rotten.

After that I spent the day relaxing with Shelly, watching DVDs. It was exactly what the both of us needed.

Monday, 27 June: (Week 25, weight; 31 stone)

So, here it is, I am down by ten stone, 140lbs. I thought I would feel a lot more excited by this but it feels paltry compared to the other stuff that is going on in my life.

Shelly rang Cork for the results and there was a problem with mine. According to the person on the phone, our blood samples were not labelled correctly and mine has gone missing. I can't understand how that happened, since we both stood and watched the doctor's receptionist label both jars in front of us. It means I have to do it all over again and race back to Cork.

I called into the parents' and ended up drafting Dad's speech, as father of the bride, for Orla's wedding. He couldn't work out how to write down what he wanted to say.

Tuesday, 28 June:

I went to Motivation, today, to be weighed and mentioned that I was coming off the diet, for a few days, on account of the wedding. One of the staff was quite put out, asking me why I taking so many days and was it really the right decision. I was well pissed off by the time I left!

Had my bout of three different sessions, swimming, working out with Chris and then a private boxing class.

Orla dropped off her dog, Roxy, today. We're going to mind her for the next three weeks which will be great company for Kerry.

Shelly had to go to the wedding rehearsal tonight.

Wednesday, 29 June:

I weighed myself and am down 141lbs. The plan was to come off the diet tomorrow but I'm feeling so fed up I just thought, **Fuck it!** Not that I went mental on it, or anything like that. All I did was eat a bowl of Crunchy Nut Cornflakes. That was it.

Dad showed me his wedding speech again. We tweaked it a bit and he should be fine now.

Ha! I double-checked what I am wearing on Friday. The shirt and the pants are fine ... but I can't wear the suit jacket because it is too big on me!

Thursday, 30 June:

Day 1 off diet: I had a white bread sandwich and, my God, did I pay for it. My stomach was in bits for hours, swollen up like an air balloon. No surprise, considering I haven't touched white bread in five months. I suppose I am going to have to be a bit careful about what I chose to eat.

I trained with Chris at 4pm, and it was hell. He is an amazing trainer. I'm convinced he must have been a Nazi in a past life.

Everything is a bit crazy here with the wedding tomorrow.

Friday, 1 July:

Day 2 off diet, and Orla's big day.

I took Nicole off for a while, in the morning, to get her away from the madness. We went to Smyth's Toy Shop where I spoilt her rotten. I dropped her back to the madness and then headed home to get myself ready.

Shelly looked absolutely gorgeous in her dress! Orla really surprised me. I had expected her to be crazy, but she was very relaxed and she looked amazing. Nicole was beautiful in her dress and so excited. They were a good half-hour late for the church. James looked mighty relieved when they finally arrived.

It was a brilliant day. I spent most of it looking after Nicole, she makes me laugh constantly.

I gave up sometime after 2am, after a lot of cider and some shots. (Obviously I am not writing this at the right time!)

Saturday, 2 July:

Day 3 off diet. I was a bit groggy this morning but we were up early, fetched Nicole, and headed down for the hotel breakfast, something I was very much looking forward to. It was a buffet so I did the only decent thing, and had a small bit of everything and it would be fair to say that it was the best breakfast I've had in a long time!

The family hung around the hotel for a while, rehashing the previous day, and then drove home to shower and get dressed for the 'after-Wedding party' in Greenhill's Hotel, commencing at 3pm. It was a relaxing day. We mostly sat out in the sun, imagining that we were in Spain. I just had the one drink, which I was perfectly happy with.

Sunday, 3 July:

Day 4 off diet. I got up early because I had to get Orla and James to the airport, for 6.30am, to fly off on their Cyprus honeymoon. Thank goodness I gave myself extra time to ring and ring and ring their phone before one of them woke up to answer me.

Later on I heard that Nicole was devastated when Orla left so I called up to take her swimming.

Thank God family weddings are not a frequent occurrence because I'm absolutely wrecked. I really should have gone back on my diet today but I am feeling slightly unmotivated. One more day can't hurt. Thinking about my food intake, of the past few days, I am pleased to say that I did not go mad, in fact I was much better than I expected myself to be, yet my poor system is completely out of whack, with the onslaught of a variety of ingredients and substances I hadn't tasted in months.

I just weighed myself: I am up by ten pounds in just four days.

This is bloody depressing.

Monday, 4 July: (Week 26, weight; 150lbs)

So I am up twelve pounds. This is so unfair; I mean, I didn't exactly let myself loose on tonnes of fattening food.

Today was about getting back to normal. I surprised myself this morning by feeling relieved to be back on track. After consuming stuff like potatoes, bread and alcohol I was lethargic and bloated. I have a feeling that this is going to be a tough week, chasing my tail in order to rid myself of the extra twelve pounds.

Nevertheless I am proud of myself for staying in control. The thing about the severity of my diet is that my body was always going to have a strong reaction the first time I touched carbohydrate or sugar since starting it. I had been warned that the smallest intake would result in immediate weight gain and also I would feel it myself, which I certainly did in terms of feeling bloated, being full of wind, and lacking in energy. The interesting thing was how things tasted different to me, for instance I found milk to be really sweet. Despite letting myself lose, for the wedding, I sort of stuck to eating healthier food, like fruit, because it was way more enjoyable and I could taste it better.

Tuesday, 5 July:

I was back in Motivation today. My weight is up ten pounds, though a lot of this was water retention. This is the downside of the ketosis diet, when you have any kind of carbohydrates the body's reaction is to pull in water. It has been explained to me that it is similar to how a woman's weight varies during the menstrual cycle. So I had known to expect this but it is a completely different thing to get on the scales and see a ten-pound gain. No matter how much I might have expected it, it was still shocking to have it confirmed.

Unfortunately, Siobhan, my usual consultant, and the one who I feel really gets me, was on holidays. I wish someone had told me because I much prefer to be dealt by someone who knows my story. It's disjointing to have a new person asking me questions I have already answered.

Afterwards I had a tough work-out with Chris. My arm was sore from boxing so we had to work around it. Chris decided we would concentrate on my flexibility, which turned out to be sore. In order to test me, he had me stretch to the point of pain, to stretch my nerves that were poor on flexibility, from the back of my knees down to my toes. I have to admit that, as painful as it was, I felt brilliant when we were finished.

Wednesday, 6 July:

By 10am I had seen the dentist, for a filling, signed on at the Dole Office and had my monthly blood tests done for my diet, to make sure being in ketosis wasn't affecting my kidneys or liver.

Friday, 8 July:

I was feeling good this morning but it only lasted until I went out to clean the shed, in the back garden, and hurt my sore arm lifting stuff around.

There are three banks that I have to deal with, over the debt from the fallout from my company. Two of them are grand while the third is the complete opposite to the other two. Unfortunately that was the bank that I tried to get a meeting with today, about the mortgage. The way they deal with me, ignoring my calls, putting off giving me answers, is utterly humiliating. The whole situation with them makes me so angry, not that it gets me anywhere.

I struggled with the diet today so I went and got some steak for my dinner, just for a change, which helped just a little. It does get difficult on the diet when I am stressed about other stuff. I suppose I am still in the progress of breaking my reliance on my old friend – food – when things get tough.

Sunday, 10 July:

I went along to the club to help out, because I still wanted to be part of it. At one point I felt really gutted about missing the fight; the atmosphere in the dressing rooms was electric.

It was busy day and by the end of it I was wrecked. Then, I'm not quite sure how it happened but someone handed me a pint and I began drinking it, completely forgetting about the diet. By the time I remembered it I was almost finished, so I just thought, **Ah fuck it!** I ended up having a couple more with the lads, which messes up the diet.

Monday, 11 July: (Week 27)

A busy day today! There was another charity event for the boxing tonight and tomorrow the family and I are off to England.

This morning I decided that I might as well have a few drinks tonight since I had some last night, so does it really matter? As soon as I thought that I got freaked, unsure that I was just making a decision for tonight or was I giving in for good?

In any case, I had one of the best nights out, drinking more than my fair share. But, Jesus, it was wonderful to relax, have a laugh and, dare I say, feel normal. It was a sort of Kangaroo Court event and I was asked to be the Judge. The place was crammed with people so I was a bit surprised that I agreed immediately and, quite happily, got up in front of everyone. That is certainly one thing about the diet that is important to me; it has given me confidence to do stuff like that. Months earlier I might not even have come along never mind get up on the stage.

Limerick Charity Boxing raised a grand total of €21,000!

Tuesday, 12 July:

We were up early to fly to London. All the way up I was dreading squeezing into a Ryanair plane, but it wasn't too bad, all things considered.

I am glad we are going away for a few days as it should help me get back on track with the diet, as well as giving my arm, along with the rest of me, a break from the training. We're staying with my aunt Aileen and hired a car to get to her place, where we just chilled out for a few hours.

In the afternoon we drove out to Virginia Water Park, which reminded me of Dublin's Phoenix Park. There are trees from all over the world, which was cool, it is also the park mentioned in Ruth Fields book **Run Fat Bitch Run** and seeing how beautiful it is made me see how easy it was for her to run there every day. On the way back to the car, Shelly and I were a good bit ahead of the others so I took the opportunity to have a little jog down the road and was very happy with myself!

Wednesday, 13 July:

We all went to Legoland today, including Aileen and her eight-year-old grand-daughter, Katie, who is great company for Nicole. I even got on the roller-coaster, something I would not have dared to, all those months ago, and completely forgot about myself too.

The other thing I forgot was my food; I left it in Aileen's house. So I had to have fruit and a sandwich, which was healthy enough, but still it fucks up the diet, which I seem to be doing a lot lately. Seriously, though, I am getting pissed off with myself and the diet. I hate feeling that I might go out of control.

Aside from that hiccup, it was a brilliant day. My legs are wrecked with all the walking we did, so at least I am staying very active.

Thursday, 14 July:

Chilled out today and I was back on track with the diet. Thank God!

Sunday, 17 July:

Wow! I am on the diet six months today. I can't decide if it feels like a long time or like it has been just a few weeks. Anyway, the important thing is that I am completely back on track with it, and I am feeling good, both emotionally and mentally. Those few days away were needed even more than I realised.

I'm a bit worried about going on Ray's show this week because I will only be about minus 9.5stone, instead of where I should be, well over ten stone. As hard as I try to stay positive it is something I'm fretting about. My feeling is that I have not just let myself down but everyone else too. Siobhan emailed me to confirm I'm on air, on Wednesday, so Shelly is going to come with me for moral support.

Shelly brought Nicole down to her Mam's in Tipperary to collect the dog. I stayed here to catch up on a few things, including this diary. I guiltily read over the last month of 'diot breaks' and am determined not to be distracted by another thing. Next month I want to be down two stone!

Monday, 18 July: (Week 28)

I had to get a new phone today so I treated myself to an iPhone. When I got back into the car, I put on the radio and guess what Ray D'Arcy was talking about … iPhones. Spooky! I pretty much spent the rest of the day trying to work out how to use the bloody thing. I thought they were meant to be easy to use.

Right, I have sorted myself out once more. It is okay to have taken two steps back so now I pick myself up again and move forward. My big goal, at the moment, is to be under thirty stone by my birthday, 19 August. I might as well face up the fact that whatever number comes up on Wednesday, when they weigh me on air, I will need to lose around two stone for next month. The important thing is to stay motivated, forget about last month and concentrate on next month instead. And that's that!

Tuesday, 19 July:

Shelly doesn't know it but she's going to be coming on air with me tomorrow. Siobhan emailed to ask me if she would be prepared to do it. I doubt she would if I gave her time to think about it so I've just told her that she will be watching me from outside the studio, and I've deleted Siobhan's email, just to be safe.

We will be having an early night tonight because of our 5am start tomorrow morning.

Wednesday, 20 July:

The alarm went off at 4.30am. I should have set it for 3.30am because Shelly took ages to get ready, making us late getting on the road. Although I have to admit it was worth it since she looked fantastic. We easily made it to Dublin and I got parking right beside Digges Lane by 8am.

We went into Today FM, for 9am, and were met by Siobhan, who asked Shelly how she was feeling about going on air. Poor Shelly's face was priceless and it was impossible for her to say no. Siobhan asked me if I was okay to talk about that day in school, with the substitute teacher. I was reluctant as I wasn't sure I could discuss it without breaking down. It shocks me how emotional I still get whenever I think about it. This is the only thing I have ever said

'no' to talking about on air; even writing about it is hard enough
as I can still see his face as if he's on front of me.

Siobhan brought us down to the studio and introduced Shelly
to Ray, Jenny and Mairead who were absolutely wonderful in
welcoming her. The interview went well apart from weighing
457lbs, which was a disappointment. I hate making excuses, but
between money worries, being out of work, and the fertility clinic
stuff my head just isn't a hundred per cent focused on losing
weight. It was great for Shelly to what happens in the studio.
We both talked about what has been happening regarding the
fertility clinic. It was probably a bit off topic, regarding the diet,
but it is hugely relevant to the big picture of why I am doing this.

At some point I accidentally blurted out that I was thinking
about doing the marathon, or, at least, thinking about giving it a
go. It has been something that has been sitting in the back of my
head for the last couple of weeks but I didn't think I was ready to
say it out loud yet.

Before we left, Ray gave me a signed copy of Gerry Duffy's
book, **Who Dares, Runs**, which is about how Gerry lost four stone,
gave up smoking and ran thirty-two marathons in thirty-two
consecutive days around Ireland, in other words, a story about
complete transformation. The man himself had written a lovely
message of support inside the cover. I was very touched. The book
could prove very inspiring if I am serious about the marathon.

On the way home, we stopped in at Shelly's Mam, in Tipperary,
and Shelly ended up staying there, and will get the train back
tomorrow or Friday. I got back here after 6pm and was exhausted.

It has been a great day. I am so thrilled that Shelly got to be a part of the show today; she has been my rock throughout.

In late July or early August I made out a 'bucket list' of goals and I looked at the list and thought, 'Where do I start with this?' I remember quietly mentioning it the Chris one day in training and tentatively asking him if he thought I could do the Dublin City Marathon. Without a second thought he smiled and replied, 'Sure, mate. Let's do it!' From this moment on, Chris became more than a personal trainer, he became my friend. Only a friend will go the extra mile and Chris was willing to do 26.2 of them with me.

So in August Chris and I started to adapt my training schedule to help me achieve my goals. We were just getting into a rhythm when I started college; due to my new schedule, we had to change my training times, so after a few weeks Chris invited me to join his 5pm class in the gym. I agreed, with some trepidation. In any case I turned up for the first session and met my new classmates. There were about a dozen of us, all shapes and sizes; some were just interested in losing weight while others were training for big stuff like the Ironman competitions, triathlons and marathons. To my relief they were all very welcoming and supportive about what I was doing. I'm not sure why this surprised me because in general I find sports people to be very accepting and encouraging, which is such a massive help.

Over the weeks and months I noted how my fitness level was improving as I did my best to keep up with these guys. I turned up early for training, and was fiercely competitive. For instance, if they did fifteen reps (repeats), I did sixteen. It was the only way I could do this, push myself to be better than them in the hope that I might, some day, be as good as them.

The more I fell in love with my new lifestyle the less effort was required to work at it. As I was losing weight I was growing in confidence. With every stone I lost I was also losing the emotional baggage that came with it, and was far heavier than a pound of fat. The boost in confidence led me to face my fears and go back to college, in September 2011, a particular achievement that I've very proud of. Education is an investment and I know it can open up a lot of doors for me, the potential to provide another life change in itself.

Thursday, 21 July:

I was in the pool bright and early this morning. Then, I met Chris for a workout at 2.30pm. I decided to test the water and ask him if he thought I would be able for a marathon. He surprised me by replying immediately, 'No problem, mate, it will be tough but I'll do with you'. So, that's that. I am doing the Dublin City marathon in October!

It is hours later and I'm still trying to digest my latest decision. The way I figure it is that I am testing myself. I know I can do it. Okay, so I'll only be walking it but a 42km walk is not to be sneezed at. I think it might be best to keep this one quiet for a bit, as some people might think I'm mad, since marathons are for the seriously athletic. But if I do it I can prove that anyone can do it, and just about anything else too. Plus, it gives me another good personal goal to work towards.

Friday, 22 July:

Score! I got a three-month free membership today for the gym at UL (University of Limerick), so I can start swimming there. Chris is going to be my swim coach and do stroke correction classes with me ahead of the i3 Swim, in September.

Saturday, 23 July:

I don't have much to say about today, other than I did some cleaning and went swimming.

In the afternoon I spent ages, on YouTube, watching inspirational stuff like **The Biggest Loser** and various sports bits, including the Derek Redmond piece. I find watching these kinds of things help keep me motivated.

Sunday, 24 July:

We both went swimming, this morning, in JJBs. After that we cleaned the house. Sundays just feel like every other day when you are on the dole.

Monday, 25 July: (Week 29)

I felt pretty flat this morning but I usually do, just after the radio show. The next appearance seems so far away that I struggle with my motivation level.

We went to the bank again, about the mortgage. Still nothing sorted. They really do not have a clue about ordinary people.

Chris gave me a monster workout this afternoon. He doesn't hang around. We did strength and conditioning exercises that he normally uses with tri-athletes. They are especially designed to develop your endurance, speed and core strength.

Our plan is to walk the marathon in under seven hours, as that is the time limit, something I hadn't realised. Therefore I need to average 1km every ten minutes, which is doable, I think.

I treated myself and had salmon for dinner.

Tuesday, 26 July:

Shelly and I got our bloods done, again, for the fertility clinic and brought them to Cork. D-Day is approaching, 18 August, when we meet the specialist in Cork who will tell us, I hope, exactly what the problem is. Half of me is dreading his news while the other half is excited about finally knowing what is wrong.

Wednesday, 27 July:

I went to JJBs, this morning, but had neither the energy nor the interest to do much.

Shelly's dole was cut off for no apparent reason. When she went in about it they said her file was on review as she is being switched from 'Back to Education Allowance' to 'Job Seekers' Benefit'. They never gave us any warning and, naturally, could not tell us when it would be sorted out. I seriously do not need this pressure.

AAAARRRRGGGHHHHH! Need I say more!!!!

I had a workout with Chris which did not improve my mood.

Thursday, 28 July:

I spent most of today thinking about where to go from here. I haven't heard a thing from the colleges I applied to, so I will have to start looking at other options.

My mind is just racing with ideas, plans, trying to look ahead. I wish it would slow down as it is stressing me. One idea that I am thinking about, I am almost afraid to write about it, but I was wondering about me becoming a coach, or a personal trainer. I would love to help people like me. But maybe it is far too soon to be thinking that I could help someone else?

Shelly is gone to look at a golden Labrador puppy in Clonmel.

Well, she has just arrived back and introduced me to Molly, who is very, very cute but I know only too well that the house is about to be seriously wrecked. Ah, well!

Friday, 29 July:

I went swimming this morning in the UL's fifty-metre pool. I couldn't settle, finding the bigger size and depth off putting. It was also colder than the JJBs pool.

Saturday, 30 July:

I assumed that the UL pool would be very busy on a Saturday morning so I went to JJBs instead. Afterwards I drove over to Atlantic Homecare to buy some plants for Shelly. She was delighted with them, and with me helping her in the garden, something the old me could never have done just because it would have been physically impossible.

In the evening I watched loads of re-runs of **The Biggest Loser**. According to the presenter a whopping 90 per cent of the contestants put back on the weight that they lose on the show. I swear that is not going to be me. I could never, ever go back to what I was. Never!

Sunday, 31 July:

Shelly and I planned to go swimming in UL, but when we arrived at 10am it wasn't open so we went back to JJBs. Then we headed back to Atlantic Homecare and bought more plants. They have some great bargains on at the minute.

We were out in the garden all day, until 9pm, planting what we bought. The weather was gorgeous and, much more importantly, Shelly was happy.

Monday, 1 August: (Week 30)

I have to get more bloods done for Cork as there was some problem with the last batch, so I'll do it tomorrow. Today, however, I am going to enjoy a lazy bank holiday.

Tuesday, 2 August:

The pool in UL was pretty busy this morning, making me feel self-conscious for the first time in ages. I find fifty metres a bit long too, but I suppose I will get used to it. Maybe it's the fact that it is a university pool makes me a bit nervous. Whatever it is, I end up thinking fondly of my comfort zone in JJBs.

I'm booked in for a sperm test in the fertility clinic next week, which is freaking me out!

Wednesday, 3 August:

Okay, so I took the easy option and went swimming in JJBs.

Because of the bank holiday I had just one session with Chris this week. He told me that Gerry Duffy is coming to the gym in a few weeks to give a talk, and invited me to come along. I said yes but now I'm not sure. I feel like I did in Cork, like I would end up standing out of the crowd of 'normal' people. Jesus! That's not good. I feel really low.

I was looking around for courses on personal training or something along those lines, that would qualify me to work with people like myself, but there are a lot of Mickey Mouse courses out there. It is hard to decide which angle I should be focusing on.

Thursday, 4 August:

Shelly took Molly to the vet this morning because she was sick, and, I suppose, after our experience with Becky, Shelly is understandably nervous. They are doing tests so we will just have to wait and see.

I received an email from Jenny, in Today FM. Ray is on holidays so my appearance has been pushed back from 17 to 31 August. While I am happy enough to postpone because, as far as I'm concerned it means that Ray does actually want me on **his** show, while he is there, I was just getting into the two week build to being weighed on air and the interview. Now, as I sit here the 31st seems like ages and ages away, and I just feel ugghh, what's the point!

We finally got something sorted out with the bank and our mortgage payments, although I'm still annoyed as apparently the decision was made weeks ago but no one thought to contact us and put our minds at rest. Typical!

At this stage I just want to see the back of thirty stone. I'm withered by it and everything else at the moment. I feel angry this week, I seem to be continually stressing about the future and so on.

Friday, 5 August:

Day 1 of my abstinence from sex, ahead of this Monday's sperm test.

I was in UL pool this morning. Chris will start coaching me there next week so I want to work on feeling comfortable in it. It is so big, so open and there are always far too many people around, so I end up feeling the old self-consciousness again, which depresses me, making me worry that I'm going backwards instead of onwards and upwards.

This afternoon I did an interview with Donal, a local journalist, from the **Limerick Leader**. He got me talking about how the diet has given me some control over my life when everything else seems so fucked up. This is so true; I just hadn't really looked at it that way, until now.

First day of abstinence and all I can think about is sex!

Saturday, 6 August:

Day 2 of abstinence from sex.

Molly is still at the vets, they haven't found out what is wrong and Shelly is up the walls about her.

Gave UL a miss and went to JJBs for my swim.

I watched the Derek Redmond clip over and over again today. I find it hugely inspiring which got me thinking about the fact that quite a few people have described me as inspiring too, but, for the life of me, I don't know how anyone could be inspired by me.

Oh why, oh why, am I obsessing about sex! It would be funny if it wasn't really, **really** bloody frustrating.

In the words of Freddy Mercury, 'Don't stop me now, I'm having a good time'! Fuck them all! Nothing and nobody is going to stop me from reaching seventeen stone, not the dole, not the bank, they can all go swing!

Saturday, 7 August:

Day Three of abstinence from sex.

It was a day with DVDs and taking it easy with Shelly. Well, the DVDs were to take my mind off tomorrow, which is stressing me out. They had to be action films too, to take my mind of sex as well as my fear about the test.

I feel huge 'down there' … I think I'm cracking up.

Monday, 8 August: (Week 31)

Now I am just back from Cork where I can honestly say I had the weirdest day of my life to date, just the most bizarre experience of my life. Firstly, the second someone tells you not to have sex, like any red-blooded male with a beautiful wife you can only think of one thing, so for days I had been thinking about sex.

So I walked into CFC and up to the reception desk where the receptionist was amazingly discreet and put me at complete ease, but considering what I was about to do it was still pretty weird! After filling out forms I was asked to wait in the waiting room, which had around fourteen people in it, all couples and all, like us, undergoing some form of fertility treatment. So it is fair to say everybody else in the room had at some stage undergone what I was about to, which probably made it worse as when I was called you could see the smiles. I was shown into the room by the receptionist. I was mortified, but she spoke as if it was nothing, told me what I had to do and left the room.

Time seemed to stand still and it took me a while to get started. Upon leaving the room I opened the door and I could see the people in the waiting room looking back at me. It's very funny, but it was very embarrassing and something I never want to have to do again.

Tuesday, 9 August:

I had an easy swim in JJBs this morning since I start with Chris tomorrow in the UL pool, which I know only too well won't be easy at all.

My afternoon was spent applying for lots of jobs. I spent €40 on printing out CVs, envelopes and postage. I bet I don't get a reply from any of them. I am seriously considering getting out of

Limerick. When is it going to get better?

Wednesday, 10 August:

So my swimming session with Chris showed me that what I have been doing and the lengths I have been swimming, for the last few months, has been nothing in comparison to this.

First, he needed to see me swim so that he could get a measure of where I was at. After that he went through lots of different moves that pieced together to form the stroke I will be using. Then there was the test, to see if I could swim the length of the pool with the new stroke. I did my best to try and remember everything but I was not prepared to look down and see Chris swimming beneath me so that he could watch my every move. I lost it from that point and was all over the place. He has given me a few exercises to work on for the next sessions.

I got home and rested a bit before going back out again, this time for the workout in the gym with Chris. I am wrecked!

We finally got Molly back this afternoon; she had 'parvo', whatever that is, some sort of virus disease. Anyway, she is on the mend, although the vet said it could take a few weeks before she'd be back to her old self.

Friday, 12 August:

I had to buy new runners today, for training and the marathon. Chris told me they were essential and only to be worn for training. They were €100, the most I have ever spent on shoes, so I hope they are worth it.

Sweet Mother of God! I have just got off the phone with the fertility clinic; they need me to do yet **another** sperm test. Apparently my results were very good in comparison to the test I did two years ago, here in the hospital in Limerick. The difference is significant and they want to be sure that no mistake has been made. I've to do it next week, when Shelly and I come in for our consultation.

Saturday, 13 August:

The UL pool is closed for the weekend due to some big competition they are holding, so I had to go JJBs. Now that I have gotten used to UL, my old pool feels too small for me. Never thought I'd be writing that.

I spent the afternoon online, researching courses.

Monday, 15 August: (Week 52)

Back to abstaining from sex until Thursday.

Training with Chris was brilliant today. We did a circuit that specifically focuses on strength and conditioning for a marathon. There was plenty of movement: squats; jumps; deadlifts; sprints and so on. I did a full fifty-six minutes without a break which was good going. We start running outside on Wednesday. Yikes!

Gerry Duffy's talk is tomorrow. Chris mentioned it to me again. I don't know what to do. I thought I had come on so much but I do feel, confidence-wise, that I am back to square one again. The audience are going to be made up of fifty triathletes and marathon runners – in other words not one of them are going to be overweight or look anything like me, or be as poor as me. Fuck! I thought I had dealt with this sort of stuff; it has just crept up on me.

Tuesday, 16 August:

I am feeling shit, tired, run down and I think my tonsils are starting to act up again.

Well, I didn't go to the Gerry Duffy talk. I didn't want to be the large, pink elephant in a roomful of serious athletes. I'm not sure that I made the right decision. Okay, I know I didn't make the right decision. I feel really bad about it, I've let myself down and I even feel that I've let Chris down.

Wednesday, 17 August:

Chris and I officially started our marathon training this morning. I met him at 7am, in the UL pool, for swimming instruction, and then we went out to the pitches for some interval training. He had me run for one minute, walk for three minutes, and so on, making sure my heart rate stayed at 145bpm (beats per minute). I enjoyed the running though I was a bit tired from the tough swim class.

So, tomorrow is the big day. Shelly and I will find out whether we can have children or not. It is strange to think that the information will mean absolutely nothing to anyone else, but the whole world to the two of us. I think I have accepted that I won't father a child. However, if they told us that we couldn't have IVF or any other fertility treatment, I honestly don't know how I would be, and I would be very, very worried about Shelly having to cope with this sort of news. I feel so tense and worried as I write this.

Thursday, 18 August:

This has been one of the greatest days in my life!

Shelly and I drove to Cork, where I had to go make a 'sample', which proved difficult when my phone started ringing at a crucial point. It was difficult not to giggle with Shelly when we went to sit in the waiting room, with everyone knowing what I had been doing. Fortunately, though, it wasn't as busy this time. We had to fill out loads of paperwork and then we met with the specialist who talked us through everything.

Shelly was taken off to be examined and when she came back the doctor gave us the medical diagnosis of 'No Medical Reason'. There was no medical reason for not getting pregnant. My heart sank at this but he rushed to assure me that this was a good thing, a very good thing indeed. It means that my sperm is perfectly normal and Shelly is perfectly normal too. It took me a while to understand this. For so long I have believed that my sperm was useless and that we would only have a baby with IVF. Now this man was telling my sperm was fine and we didn't need IVF. He told us our chance of getting pregnant was high, if we got some IUI, and we can get that for free.

In other words, by this time next year, Shelly could well be pregnant.

I don't think it has fully sunk in yet.

Our next step is Shelly having to get a HGC scan, where dye

will be injected into her womb, to check her Fallopian tubes. She has been warned that it is painful, and will cost €450, but it is a step further along the road because then we will be referred to CUMH (Cork University Maternity Hospital), who will give us four treatments of IUI, injecting my sperm into her womb, while giving her a course of drugs that will make her more fertile.

We are so happy; neither of us expected this kind of result.

Friday, 19 August:

Happy Birthday to me!

I am thirty-one years of age, and for the first time since I was eighteen, my weight is below my age … just about, at any rate. It is still too heavy. This time next year I aim to be seventeen stone or even less. All along I have said I would be happy to reach seventeen stone, but I also want to be really fit with a good muscle mass too. I'm not saying that I am hoping to have a six-pack, but I certainly wouldn't mind a hint of one. God knows it would make a very pleasant change from a keg!

I went to the doctor because I still felt rotten but he told me it was just a head cold which is good in one way, it's nothing serious, but thanks to my diet I can't take anything for it. At least, I am determined not to, I don't want my weight fluctuating again, messing around with my concentration. How many people know that most tablets are coated in sugar … okay, tiny of amounts of sugar, but still?

Mam made me a jelly birthday cake to make me feel like I am having a real birthday treat. She is so good to me.

Saturday, 20 August:

I got up at 8am and went out to UL to do a 5km walk/run, but didn't quite make it to the 5k. I think I maybe pushed a bit too hard on the running because I started to feel really nauseous. So I jumped in the car and drove to JJBs, for a quick swim. Then I went and sat in the sauna room for as long as I could bear it, in an effort to shift this cold.

Monday, 22 August: (Week 33)

Molly ate my swimming goggles so I have to wear Shelly's purple ones for a few days.

Had to take Sudafed yesterday, for the cold, and I felt the benefit of it when I woke up this morning, feeling ever so slightly better.

I was at UL for 7am, for the run/walk and then I went for a swim.

Well, I had given up on hearing anything but today CAO offered me a place on LIT's Business and Marketing Diploma/Degree course. Because I was convinced I didn't get it, and was looking around for options, I was completely unprepared. In other words now I have mixed emotions about it ... including fear. Oh, shit! What will I do?

Some months previously, I had decided I would apply to go back to college. I remember looking through some booklets in sheer bewilderment and thinking, 'What the hell will I do?' I selected a few courses on the basis of what I like the sound of and perhaps how my experiences to date could be best used. At the time I was just applying to see if I would get in; I hadn't thought about it too much as so many other things were happening so getting a place really was a surprise and while initially happy I was also terrified. I was still very heavy and the thought of going into college really was unnerving.

Tuesday, 23 August:

I went to Motivation to be weighed, and somehow I am up a whole fucking stone of water. How the fuck did that happen? I seriously felt close to tears when she told me. It is thanks to the tablets I took to treat the bloody cold, along with the hot lemon drinks. I am so, so disappointed with myself. Honest to God, I don't know what to say or think other than I am filled with an overwhelming sense that I am letting everyone down.

Wednesday, 24 August:

I had a 6.45am training session with Chris in UL. We did a 6km walk, but no running because the muscles in my legs are a bit tender with all this new exercise. After that we hit the pool at 8am for a sixty minute session that I thoroughly enjoyed. I feel so much better today, and I do believe it is the exercise that helps me to return to positive form when I've been down in the dumps.

At 3am I drove back to UL for a second swim which would have been more enjoyable had there not been a group of lads acting like assholes. I did some aqua jogging too, which was fun.

Thanks to my immense feeling of well-being today, I have decided that I am going to give college a go and see where it leads to. It is a great course and I have done well to get a place on it.

Friday, 26 August:

What a good day this has been!

Firstly I had a great session in the UL pool this morning. Then Shelly's dole was finally sorted out, which is a load off my shoulders. Our money has improved, I have made my decision about college and we are still reeling from the good news at the fertility clinic. Things are finally starting to look up for us. And, on top of all that good news, I am back down to 430lbs, so I am just ten pounds away from thirty stone.

I am now trying to sort out my grant application, to cover the college fees. There is so much paperwork involved.

Monday, 29 August: (Week 34)

I weighed myself this morning, ahead of the Ray D'Arcy Show tomorrow, and I'm 427lbs, in my boxer shorts, which is okay, I guess.

I am wondering if I should try looking for bouncer work. It is the right of the year for it; however, is it a good idea? We need the money but would I be playing with fire, both mentally and emotionally, if I returned to the negative stuff, the personal abuse that comes with the job?

Tuesday, 30 August:

I had my 7am swim in UL before heading on the road to Dublin.

When I got to Marconi House, lugging the scales in with me,

I marvelled at how completely relaxed I was. My visits to the studios almost feel ordinary to me, like getting petrol for the car or seeing the doctor.

It was a great interview. Because I was wearing clothes I weighed in at thirty-one stone, or 434lbs, so I was down one stone, which I was happy enough with. Although, I couldn't help feeling that the others, including maybe the listeners, were a bit disappointed with this. I guess, to them, one stone is only one stone, while I am just relieved to be losing weight. People are so much more excited when I lose two stone. I certainly have slowed down all right, and I'm not sure why, since I am exercising more than I ever had.

I told Ray I was going to the Dublin Marathon in October which seemed to surprise him a little, but, as usual, he was hugely supportive and, as usual, I left the studio feeling like I was on cloud nine. It is so important to be positive when someone is doing their best to improve themselves. I cannot underestimate the importance of Ray's and his team's support. They help spur me on to dream about doing things like marathons.

Wednesday, 31 August:

Back to reality after yesterday's show, this can sometimes be tricky regarding my mood and motivation levels. It is like I build myself up for the show and then, the following day, I come right back down again. However, I am determined to kick ass this month and get back on the road to losing two stone.

I had a good swim session with Chris this morning. My

technique is starting to come together and with a bit more work at sharpening it, I should be able to focus on improving my speed. After that we walked around the pitches for an hour. The walk doesn't feel as long when I have him to talk to.

I have been invited out, on Saturday night. It is Deccy's (from the boxing club) birthday and a whole bunch of the lads are going out for dinner and drinks. I want to go but I have huge reservations about sticking to the diet. Sitting with fellas tucking into chips and knocking back pints might prove to be too much of a temptation, and I know Deccy would understand that. Should I just excuse myself and stay at home?

Saturday, 3 September:

I did an 8km walk this morning before dropping Sholly into work. Then I brought Nicole swimming in UL.

So, I decided to head out, for a while, to Deccy's birthday dinner. The plan was to stay for an hour or two but I ended up staying out until 1am. I was very good, I drank water and had steak and broccoli for dinner. We were having such a good laugh I didn't miss drinking cider or having potatoes.

I had a really interesting chat with Johnny Kiely, who works with athletes. He was asking me about the diet, whether or not it was having a positive effect on my brain, was I sharper and more positive than before I started it. This was something I hadn't thought about and I was delighted he asked, because the truth is that mentally I do feel a hell of lot sharper and efficient.

Apart from having a great night, I am also delighted with the fact that I wasn't one bit self-conscious. I relaxed and enjoyed myself, just like everyone else.

Monday, 5 September: (Week 35)

Shelly started back in college this morning and then I start college next week, so my schedule is going to be up in the air for a bit.

I enjoyed an early walk at 6.30am, followed by a recovery session in the pool, which include swimming and aqua jogging.

Thursday, 8 September:

Nerves are setting in about college. Mostly I am excited about it but, at the same time, I wish I wasn't going to be the fat guy in the class. Will I get 'the look', will there be jokes made at my expense? I suppose there is no point in worrying about it. I'm really not sure how I am going to juggle training and college. I'm not going to be bored, that's for sure.

Friday, 9 September:

After my early morning walk and swim I sat down with Chris to work out how I was going to continue my training when I start college. He said that if I wasn't available in the day-time then I could join his evening classes, which are limited to eight people, who are, for the most part, tri-athletes.

I collected Shelly from work and brought her to Penneys because she needed new clothes for college. This time last year I would have stayed in the car, too afraid to go in with her, so I am delighted to write here that I happily accompanied her around the shop as she picked out what she wanted. Okay, I admit I was a little bit self-conscious but still, it is a huge improvement for me and great for the two of us to be able to go shopping as a couple.

Sunday, 11 September:

The Marathon Des Sables, in Morocco, which involves covering 243km (151 miles), through the Sahara Desert, in six days, is the toughest footrace on earth, and the equivalent of five and a half regular marathons ... and I want to do it!

It is open to people aged sixteen to seventy-eight years, with a variance in time limits, between 3 and 14km an hour, so you can do it in seven days if necessary. Competitors must carry everything they need in a backpack though water, which will be rationed, is given out at every check point. In other words I would have to carry six or seven days worth of food on my back, in temperatures reaching 120 degrees Fahrenheit, as I run/walk over terrain that includes sand dunes and rocky, uneven ground.

Incorrect shoes and equipment may be dangerous in that heat and covering that distance. I would imagine that mental stamina is just as important as physical stamina, to cope with such a demanding journey. For instance, after four days you set out bright and early to complete over forty miles across barren land. Few people complete this before it gets dark that evening. In fact, I have read that some don't make it back until the following evening. Then, when you have accomplished that, you are ready for the 42km run.

It may sound mad but if I do this, or make the serious effort to do it, I will be exactly opposite to where I was in January. I want to prove that someone like me could do something wild like this. Once people assumed that I was nothing else but a fat, lazy slob. Imagine if I could banish that assumption forever, after doing something like this.

I just need to figure out how to make it happen.

Apart from dreaming up crazy stuff to do, and to set as goals, I also did some housework and went for a swim. So, it was a good day!

Monday, 12 September: (Week 36)

I'm starting to have big reservations about college, mostly based on how it will impact on the diet and training. Registration is tomorrow at 2pm and I had thought that would be it until I start next Monday, but I have just found out that I have three orientation days, this week: Wednesday, Thursday and Friday. This means I have to mess Chris around, which is frustrating and nerve-wracking. I don't want my fitness level to drop.

Shelly is off to Cork tomorrow, for the HSG scan. Her mother is bringing her down since I have to register for college. They warned us it would be really sore, so I hope she is okay.

Tuesday, 13 September:

Okay, so college registration was a little daunting, with not one familiar face, but at least it is done. I'm going to see how the induction days go, and give it a chance. I suppose it is natural to be nervous about it, going back to college after all these years and

I'm assuming that I'll be the oldest in the class too.

I got a wetsuit sorted for Saturday's i3 Swim.

Shelly came back from Cork and said that the scan went well and that the specialist was very happy with her. Later on she experienced some soreness, comparing it to bad period pains and nothing worse.

Wednesday, 14 September:

It was a savage session in UL, this morning. Everything came together regarding technique and speed, making me feel rather chuffed with myself. You can't beat that feeling when you finally get the hang of something and it begins to feel natural. Then, as I was getting out of the pool, I was brought back to earth with a bang, when I spotted a guy giving me 'the look' of disgust. It flattened me, reminding me that I had a long way to go yet.

I spoke briefly to Chris today and asked him about the Marathon De Sables. He trained a guy to do it last year so he knows exactly what is involved. He said he would have a think about it and get back to me.

Today's induction day, at college, was never-ending. We all agreed it seemed a bit pointless after the first couple of hours. I had a bit of a moment when the first speaker put us in pairs to demonstrate how to work together. I was paired up with a woman who was a lecturer. So, when the exercise was finished, and the speaker asked for a show of hands from people who felt they had had to work with someone who was a mismatch, my partner put up her hand and the whole class laughed. A few months earlier this might have crushed me but I was actually okay about it. I just feel I'm so different now, to what I used to be like, in terms of confidence and sensitivity.

They showed us our lecture halls and, thank God, the seats are bigger than I was expecting, so that was a huge relief.

I took a quick walk this evening. It was meant to be a long walk but I made the mistake of bringing the dogs with me and they slowed me down, constantly stopping to sniff everything, so I turned around and walked them back home, in a huff.

Thursday, 15 September:

I have come to realise that I am a creature of habit, in that I dislike change, and I absolutely hate not having a schedule. Routines help people to feel they have a bit of control over their life and, right now, I feel like I am being tossed around on ocean waves. I am becoming really impatient for my college time-table to be worked out so I can sort out my training around it. In any case I will be swimming every morning at 7am, before college, which is grand as I really enjoy it.

Friday, 16 September:

After college, Shelly and I drove to Killaloe to test the wet suit for tomorrow. It was a horrible mistake! Firstly, the weather was brutal and, secondly, the water was bloody freezing. I pushed off into the water but between the cold instantly snatching my breath away, it being too dark to see where I was going, along with the creepy sensation of the wetsuit filling up with water, I panicked and got straight back out again. The whole experience threw me and, consequently, I am not looking forward to tomorrow's competition. I rang Chris and he is going to come out early with me so we can see what is happening with the wetsuit. I may have to do the swim without it.

Saturday, 17 September: (i3 open water swim, Killaloe)

Well, the weather was crap for the swim today. Chris and I drove out early to register and allow ourselves time to warm up properly. Carly, his partner, and children came out to watch us. I'm not sure how it happened but we lost track of time, probably because we were chatting so much. Suddenly the announcement for all swimmers to take their positions, at the starting line, came out over the loudspeakers. As I was pulling on the wetsuit as fast as I could, I remembered the terror of yesterday and was overcome with nerves. Chris was brilliant; he calmed me down and assured me that I was well able for it.

It was more than a little embarrassing when we copped that the race was being delayed especially for us so we told them to go ahead, explaining that neither of us were there to actually race, I was just there to do it. Once the race started I could take my time getting into the water. At the point of me submerging myself the others would have been about 150 metres ahead in the distance. Just like yesterday, the cold took my breath away but it wasn't as bad. Chris swam beside me keeping me calm, telling me to ease myself into the swim before I let myself go for it. It took me a few minutes to put my face in the water, which was still unpleasant as the water was so dark.

Chris was my guide, swimming in front of me so all I had to do was follow him; Chris actually swam the whole race backwards! I started to get into it when I could clearly see a few of the swimmers ahead of me, and it quickly dawned on me that this meant I was catching up on them. A sudden spurt of instinctive competitive spirit sent me chasing after them and, lo and behold, I passed them out. Alternating between the breast stroke and the free style I completed the half-mile race in thirty-four minutes, which I was absolutely delighted with, not least because I had beaten **four** other swimmers. I never imagined that I might actually beat anybody so this was a colossal bonus, regarding my self-confidence and sense of achievement.

When I got out of the water I was numb with the cold but then Chris and I had another challenge. Ireland was playing Australia, in rugby, and he has Sky-plussed it. All we had to do was get back to his house before we could find out the results. His phone was beeping away with text messages, as we drove along, and he had a total of twenty-five texts by the time he put the key in his front door, so we kind of reckoned Ireland had won, which they had. Great match!

We watched the match in Chris's house while Chris minded his two lovely children, Jamie and Corin. With everything that was going on with the fertility specialist, I couldn't but envy Chris playing with his two kids. I always wanted children, hopefully now we can start getting some answers. I realise it will probably be a sperm donor or some other route, but just having an option would be amazing.

Monday, 19 September: (Week 37)

First official day of my Business Management and Marketing course or at least it was after I went for my swim in UL. I am excited about it, about what it could lead to. I'm still trying to think about what I want to do with my life and to incorporate my interests or passions. Food is one of my passions, though not in the way it used to be. These days I am very passionate about the correct marketing and labelling of food, which is largely why I wanted to study marketing and find out all about it for myself. Sometimes I dream about setting up my own food label, like 'Love Irish Food', whereby any company that makes genuinely healthy food, with quality ingredients, is allowed to use a symbol on their label that promotes their 'food integrity' to the consumer, who is then making a completely informed decision about what they want to buy.

It was fair enough, we met all our lecturers but not too much done in the way of work. I'm, by far, the oldest in my class, which I expected to be. They seem like a nice bunch though. At least they don't talk about the recession; they're too young to be bothered about stuff like that. And, surprisingly enough, I have only received a couple of 'the looks'.

So these are the subjects that I will be studying this year: Management and Marketing; Principals of Economics; Accounting; Mathematics and Statistics; Enterprise Development and Business Communications; Business Technology and Office

Applications.

The one thing that worries me is the maths. I'm okay with plain old numbers but fancy stuff like algebra is a different matter. On the other hand I know that my experience, in setting up my own company, is going to be a huge help to me. I suppose it will all balance out in the end.

There is a canteen but I think I will steer clear of it. It's probably better if I bring my own lunch and eat it in the car so that I can listen to the radio. Some days I'll just come home, depending on when my next class is.

I just went out for a quick walk this evening.

Going back to college was a bit of a surprise; I had sort of given up on it, but then I figured that I had a new life with new possibilities and that a new education or path in life would be an amazing addition to everything else I was doing. Though it's vital for people, I've always found signing on very negative – most people only do it because they have to; I don't know anybody who likes having to sign on so for me it was a massive positive change.

Twelve months previously I would not have even fitted into the lecture theatre seats let alone be able to get past the psychological barriers, so going back was a massive sign of how far I had come; I now had self-belief and was eager to make the best of the person I knew I could be. I had looked at loads of courses and it was the marketing that really attracted me to this course as well as the practical side – it was based in Limerick. The course was two years with the option to do two more, so if I could not sustain it I would at least be able to hopefully get a job. Bear in mind that Shelly was going into second year in UL, so it was a strange situation with the two of us back at college.

Tuesday, 20 September:

I decided to be a bit pro-active and email my Year Head, asking what my classes are, so that I can plan my training around them. I'm slightly unsure as to whether I should mention the diet and training.

'If you do not give up, you can not fail!' I love this quote and feel that it particularly apt for me, in that the only way I won't reach my goals is if I give up, and I have absolutely no intention of doing that. The truth is I am enjoying my new life way too much to stop now.

Wednesday, 21 September:

Gillian, my Year Head, got back and invited me to meet her to discuss my situation. Fortunately she had heard me on the radio and knew my story and was very supportive about it. I think my classmates are too young to be fans of Ray; she's the first person to mention it at any rate. So she very kindly allowed me to choose, from four options, my own time-table, to accommodate the extra-curricular stuff. This is a load off my shoulders, as I hate not knowing what I am doing from day to day.

That nice chat was followed by a heavy day at college, including three hours of Economics. I feel that my brain is fried so I'm going to go out for a walk, now, to clear my head before turning in.

Thursday, 22 September:

I went for an early morning walk, at 6.30am, and then I had a quick swim and headed off to college.

Chris wants me to join his evening classes, on Monday, Wednesday and Friday, at 5pm. I feel just a little bit apprehensive, but not for the usual reason, of me being the biggest and so forth. It is just that I have heard his class is tough-going so I worry about my being able to keep up with it. Nevertheless I am chuffed that he asked me to join the class of athletes. Also I know that if he felt I couldn't do it, he wouldn't have said it to me. That's one of his best qualities, as a personal trainer, he really does wonders for my confidence.

Looking back I remember having reservations because of the people who train in Chris's classes. They are marathon runners, triathletes and Ironmen, so they really were on a very high level. Having to go into the same class as them was certainly intimidating as they were such good athletes. But in the end no one was anything but welcoming.

Saturday, 24 September:

I did a very decent 12km walk, this morning, which I enjoyed except for the blisters. It really pisses me off that I still get them, after all this exercising. You would think that my feet would be well able for anything now.

When I got home I showered and dropped Shelly into work, and had planned to go straight to the UL pool but I changed my mind. I don't know if it was just the blisters but I suddenly felt frustrated and in bad form, as if someone has poked me with a pin and all the air went rushing out of me.

Fortunately, my mood improved by the afternoon so I went for my swim which was only marginally ruined by a gang of young lads acting the gobshite!

Sunday, 25 September:

My feet were quite sore today so I went and did a great aqua jogging session in UL. In other words I turned a negative into a positive, and, in doing so, cheered myself up no end.

Monday, 26 September:

Following a long day at college I hit Chris' gym for my first 'Strength and Conditioning' group session. The others guy in the class are a really nice bunch and, though the session was as tough as I feared, I really enjoyed being part of the group.

Mentally, I feel very positive about where I am, in relation to the gym class and to college in general. It has to be a huge factor that I got myself off the dole, I really cannot think of anything worse, though I certainly kept myself busy with training. I think I feel more in control of my life and the future. Making the decision to re-train myself for a job that will help me pay off the debts, it was such a powerful positive step to take. I am only really appreciating that now. Shelly and I are much happier, individually and as a couple, with our respective courses and interests.

Wednesday, 28 September:

Oh my God, I am so tired after college today. Wednesdays are exhausting, with three hours of Economics and two hours of maths. After college I had to go for an eye test. I have been struggling to see the board in class and definitely need new glasses.

I was pissed off today. I have to get a letter from the college for my Back to Education allowance but they wouldn't give it to me since I haven't yet paid the registration fee because the VEC (Vocational Education Committee) pays that, only they won't be paying it for another few weeks. In other words it doesn't look like I'll be receiving any money next week. College said it would issue a letter but it is not going to say that I'm registered with them.

No training with Chris tonight because I had to go and have my feet seen to. The blisters are gone beyond a joke at this stage. Tauncha, the 'foot lady', has given me a regime, for the marathon. Basically, I have to bath my feet in Epsom salts and Tea Tree oil, as well as applying cream daily and using gel pads in my runners. I also have to buy a special pair of socks along with a second pair of runners so that I can alternate them, when training is intensified within the next couple of weeks.

Because of my weight I have flat feet, so they aren't the best pair of feet to be doing sports on, as the muscles are under-developed. When I told her I had to be walking–fit for the marathon in five weeks time she nearly dropped. She had been convinced up to then that I was talking about next year's marathon. I couldn't help laughing at her surprise.

Thursday, 29 September:

Well, I had an incredible start to the day. I weighed myself and found I was below thirty stone. It seems like I have been waiting such a long time to see this on the scales. Unfortunately I was home alone; I was so excited I wanted to hug someone. I wore a tee-shirt and shorts to weigh myself but when I read my weight I grabbed the camera to take a picture of the scales' reading of 419.6lbs, which meant the weight of the camera added a pound or two. Without thinking I tore off my clothes, forgetting that the curtains were open. Thank God nobody was passing; at least, I don't think anybody was.

Today, I spent €15 on a pair of socks, the most I have ever spent on socks in my life. They better work, that's all I can say!

This evening I went out for a walk, doing 7.5km in 1.07 minutes, but then I had to give up thanks to the bloody blisters. It was darker than I realised. I was on the back road to UL, which is normally quiet, and I scared the life out of a cyclist who almost collided with me because he didn't see me. I think I better get myself a Hi-Viz jacket.

Friday, 30 September:

Collected my new glasses today and then had to go into the Social Welfare with the letter from college but, just as I suspected, they won't accept it. I rang the college and tried to explain the situation again, so they are going to do me a second letter but it still won't say that I am registered with them.

I did a cross-fit circuit, at 5pm, this evening, with Chris' group.

It was tough, forty minutes straight of exercising without a break. I even got dizzy at one stage, but I didn't care. It was brilliant to be able to keep up with everyone else. After all those months of exercising alone, at home, and then one-on-one sessions with Chris, I really enjoy belonging to a group.

It struck me tonight how much Shelly and I, and our relationship has changed. It is so much better now that we are not in each other's pockets. My attitude and outlook on life is a million miles from where I was in January. For the first time in years we have quite a lot to look forward to, what with college, the fertility clinic diagnosis and my losing weight.

Saturday, 1 October:

Ha! One of the downsides of losing weight is that I am able to do housework now, which is how I spent my day. Ah well, I have to take the good with the bad, I guess.

This withers me! I went over to Xtravision to get some DVDs. It was more expensive to do what I wanted to, which was to only rent four DVDS. I had to rent the DVDS, **and** buy four cans of Coke and two tubs of popcorn, in order to avail of the special deal and get the films cheaper. I was going to dump the cans and popcorn into the bin outside but then I just brought them home and gave them to Shelly. I can do without deals like that, not that I was tempted to eat and drink the stuff; it just annoyed me that I had to buy them in order to pay less for what I wanted.

Sunday, 2 October:

I got up at 8am to watch the rugby, Ireland destroyed Italy!

Next I got ready to do a big walk, which took some preparation. In fact I want to write it down here because I can't believe the amount of stuff I have to do in order to go for a walk.

I put Vaseline under and in between my toes to prevent friction

I put on the special compression/anti-blister socks

I put gel inserts into my runners to reduce the impact against the ground

I applied Deep Heat to my knees and calves

I applied Voltarol cream to my knees and hip area

I put talk powder in my bag in case of chafing, along with two bottles of water and some euros in case I needed more water than that.

After that I was ready to rock. I did 14km in three hours and thirteen minutes which was fairly good. The aim today was to see how long I could keep walking, I didn't really care about the distance I covered.

When I got home the bad news was that my hips and knees were quite sore, but the good news was my feet were fine. All that work was worth it! I had to put ice packs on my knees for a few minutes and then I took a very, very hot shower, to relax my body. It proves to me what Chris has been saying, if I carry out the correct preparations I can do anything I want, I just have to mind myself against injury. Again, I thought about my favourite quote, 'If You Do Not Give Up, You Cannot Fail!'

Tonight Shelly and I chilled out in front of a good fire and watched a film. The pain in my hips got bad enough for me to have to take a Diphene but, apart from that, it was a pleasant, relaxing evening. That's one of the good things about all this training; it helps me to relax better when I want to, like I know I deserve it because I've worked hard.

Monday, 3 October:

My hips were still sore today but I didn't mind since I didn't have any muscle pain...or blisters. A good day, indeed!

I went for a swim at 7am and then headed into college. We started our tutorials today which meant that we have been divided up into groups of twenty, so it should make it easier to get to know a few people now.

And what a relief it was receive a dole payment today, despite the Back to Education allowance still not sorted. College gave me another letter but I know it's not going to work. What can I do but bring into the Social Welfare and hope for the best.

When I started back in college it was a double-edged sword. I was almost twelve years older than 99 per cent of the class and while they all seemed nice I was still very self-conscious and quiet. My schedule didn't help either and I probably isolated myself as I came and went so much, they didn't know anything about me and why should they? So in an effort to let my new classmates into my life, one of my lecturers suggested I tell them my story and share my experiences; it was such a massive help that the college were so supportive and wanted to help me to settle in.

Tuesday, 4 October:

It was a good day in college. The tutorials definitely help to give me a better understanding of things. Gillian, my Year Head, asked me to stay after class, which sounded ominous, but she just wanted to ask me how things were going. She also surprised me by asking if I would be interested in giving a class presentation about my diet. I wasn't sure about this but she said to think about it.

Thursday, 6 October:

So, I did think over Gillian's suggestion and told her today that I would do it. I decided to do it for two reasons. Firstly, it's an opportunity to tell my class about something that is a major part of my life so it will hopefully help me build bridges and, secondly, Gillian told me it would make an interesting talk for a marketing class. I have also been asked to give feedback to the Head of the Business Department. This is all very flattering.

I did a two-hour walk this afternoon, which went well. On the way home I called up to Mam and Dad's because it was Nicole's birthday and there was cake. I was grand about that until someone who shall remain nameless kept going on and on, and on, about how delicious the cake was!

Friday, 7 October:

I had a good swim and aqua jogging session before college this morning.

In the afternoon I had physio with Richard Rocker in Pro

Performance (advanced chiropractic centre) with a very painful, but brilliant, deep tissue massage on my lower back and legs. I felt great after it. We also discussed the diet. Richard explained about the benefit in increasing my muscle mass and losing fat, in that it will speed up my metabolism over the coming months.

This evening I trained with Chris, which went well until I was bent over in agony from ferociously-bad wind pain, making me puke and leaving me with the hiccups. The very odd side effect of weight loss is I am getting very bad trapped wind as my stomach shrinks. This means that like a baby I need to almost wind myself, which isn't very nice and very embarrassing.

Saturday, 8 October:

I got up at 5.30am to watch Ireland play Wales. Awful match! I had to go for a walk to get rid of my frustration, and did 9km in two hours. I should have walked for longer, that was the plan, but my left calf became really tight and sore. I tried stopping to stretch it but nothing worked. On the plus side my feet are good, with neither blisters nor pain. My hips are knees were fine too. I think I just have to stretch more before I start training.

Monday, 10 October: (Week 40)

So, today, I gave my presentation to the class about myself and the diet. It was introduced into a lecture about sponsorship, media and why certain companies choose to sponsor certain people, which led into a discussion on the power of the media, and, in particular, radio shows recommending products or life styles. The class were then asked by the lecturer if this sort of thing had any meaning for them and when there were no contributions, they were told that there was somebody in the room who was a regular guest on a national radio show. It was a bit daunting, but it also felt liberating to be explaining why I come and go and why I am so quiet. I spoke for about thirty minutes and answered some questions afterwards. I hope they got something from it. Overall, it was very, very positive and I am happy I did it.

Tuesday, 11 October:
An early start this morning, for my monthly weigh-in on air, in Today FM. I really enjoy it; it's almost like catching up with old friends.

The interview was brilliant, as usual, and dominated by talk about the marathon. Ray seems very concerned about my doing it. I think he is mostly worried that, if something happened to prevent me from finishing it, it might affect my motivation and confidence, which I appreciate as I believe his concern comes straight from the heart. I love hearing the listeners' reactions too, everyone is always very supportive. Sitting in the studio today, I felt really lucky to be able to avail of all this enthusiasm for my sporting ambitions.

I made it back to Limerick in time for my afternoon classes.

It was a nice part of my relationship with Ray and the show to know that Ray was concerned as it also showed he cared. I can understand his concern as I was thirty stone at the time and marathons are such a huge undertaking even for healthy and fit people.

Wednesday, 12 October:

Since I missed swimming, yesterday morning, it was good to be back in the pool today. It really is such a great way to start to start the day.

We have been put on the waiting list for CUMH (Cork University Maternity Hospital), to see if we can get the IUI treatment. Shelly spoke to them; it could take ten months for us to meet with a specialist, unless there is a cancellation. So Shelly said we would happily take a cancellation if one came up, I am not expecting anything, but who knows.

Friday, 14 October:

Only a few weeks to go, until the marathon, and I must say I am really pleased with how my training is going. My feet are holding up well so I just need to keep doing what I'm doing.

I emailed Siobhan Hogan, at Today FM, to ask her to recommend a hotel near the finish line as I don't want to have to walk much on top of the marathon. She replied and said that the station would organise the hotel for me, which is a big relief. They also want me in the studio, on the Tuesday after the marathon. I'm delighted about this. There is no way that I am not going to complete the race now that I know that I have to go and talk about it, with Ray, the very next day.

College finished at 1pm so I went for a short walk before some fairly intensive training this evening.

Monday, 17 October: (Week 41)

Two weeks to the marathon now. I'm starting to get excited about it; it's all I can think about.

I'm sure that some people think, or will think, that I am mad for doing it, but this sort of attitude just makes me more determined to take part. Of course, my family were very surprised when I first told them I was considering doing the marathon but they rallied around me immediately, and are one hundred per cent supportive. I know I can't expect everyone to react the same way. Maybe I'm wrong but I really feel that I have so much that I want to prove to other people, though I think the person I want to prove it to the most is me. Taking my place on the start line is going to be a test in itself. Will I feel comfortable or will I feel nervous and out of place?

It is time to start planning the finer points of the day, such as my running gear and deciding what I need to bring. I'm like a kid getting ready for his first day of school, with little or no idea what to expect.

Tuesday, 18 October:

Seriously, my life is all about the marathon these days.

I was contacted by a journalist from the **Sunday World**, who had gotten my details from Will Hanafin at Today FM, and wanted to do a piece about me for this weekend's paper. I enjoyed it. She was really professional and it gave me a chance to start at the beginning of this year and talk about everything that has happened up to now.

For tonight's walk, I strode into town and back home again. It is a bit of a pressure with all the training and my college work. There simply aren't enough hours in the day.

Okay, so I need to decide about my nutrition for the race. Do I stick with just protein or do I eat carbohydrates? It is a tough decision to make. If I stay on the diet and then something happens and I can't physically finish the marathon, I'm always going to be wondering what if I had eaten carbs instead. On the other hand I dislike the idea of breaking with the diet. I'm really torn.

Today FM have booked me into the Davenport Hotel, which is only about fifty metres from the finish line. Perfect!

Thursday, 20 October:

I met with the Motivation doctor this morning and asked him should I stay on the diet or not, for the marathon. His advice was to break it and eat carbohydrates, but is going to double check this with Motivation.

Shelly rang my phone when I was in class this afternoon and since I couldn't answer it, I text her, feeling sure that something was up. She would never ring when I'm in college. It turns out that CUMH rang her and said if we could get to Cork by 2pm we could have a cancellation appointment, and jump the ten month waiting list. The time was 12.10pm and I felt it was a long shot. Nevertheless, I left the lecture, raced across town to pick her up and drove to Cork like a mad thing. We made it down by 2.20pm and were hugely relieved to find that the specialist was running late, in other words we had made it on time after all. We filled out more forms, and met with the specialist who duly approved us for two treatment of IUI, to start next year. It is the best luck we have had in ages and ages.

What a day!

Friday, 21 October:

Since I didn't get out walking last night I walked for thirty minutes on UL's running track before my swim, which was far from enjoyable thanks to a dark and wet morning.

We're both over the moon from yesterday.

In the afternoon I had another physio appointment with Richard Rocker who gave me a badly needed rub down. I asked his opinion on my big carbohydrates question, for the marathon, and he emphasised that if I did choose to eat them, I was to keep it to very small amounts or else I could end up with an upset stomach and/or having the runs – no pun intended!

Sunday, 23 October:

Shelly got up early to run out and buy a copy of the **Sunday World**. Much to my relief, it was a well-written article, and I was delighted with it.

I headed out early this morning for my last long walk before the marathon, and did twenty kilometres in four hours and it wasn't without some drama. Imagine, I got pulled up by a garda, for walking in a cycle lane. He told me I had to walk on the river path, which is broken and uneven. Apart from that, it was a good walk with minor joint pain, though my feet were a little swollen. However, I was really pleased as I'm exactly where Chris had physically prepared me to be.

My right foot feels a bit sore now. I did the whole ice bath and foot bath routine so hopefully it will be better by tomorrow.

Monday, 24 October: (Week 42)

I feel so excited, as if it was Christmas, because it is just one more week to the marathon. I had my usual swim, before college, with some aqua jogging and stretching. Okay, I am slightly worried about my right foot. It doesn't feel right. In fact it feels to me like there is something moving around inside of it. It's not sore, just feels weird, but maybe it is just a little stiff.

Ray D'Arcy wants to interview me on Thursday, by phone, in a sort of panel discussion that includes Johnny Donnelly (marathon runner, formerly of the band, the Saw Doctors) and Gerry Duffy. Now, I'm not sure how much help I will be, in comparison to the two guys, but I am flattered to have been invited to contribute.

Tuesday, 25 October:

Roll on next Monday, that's all I can say. Except for my foot I feel bloody amazing and cannot wait to take my place at the starting line.

I went to see my own doctor today. He checked my blood

pressure and my heart, and everything is fine. When I asked him about the diet he said, rather bluntly, 'You wouldn't try to drive to Dublin on €20 worth of fuel, would you?' I shook my head and he continued, 'So, you also need the right amount of fuel to run a marathon'.

My foot is still giving me trouble. I walked for an hour tonight and not once could I forget about it. All I can do is keep icing it, giving it Epson Salt foot baths and massaging it. I wish the rest of my body was as well looked after.

Thursday 27th October

So today was the first time I really thought hang on a second something isn't right here while in with Motivation, you may have noticed I don't mention them much and that is because for some time I have felt a little messed around by them since my original consultant left Motivation Limerick.

Anyway it is fair to say we have had ups and downs, but the results spoke for themselves so I just put on a smile and went with it, but today I was very taken aback. I realise what I am doing – the marathon is very extreme but they have said that I am to stay on the diet which is in stark contrast to what two doctors have said, I told my consultant this and the response just made no sense so I am genuinely frustrated and confused and really feel like enough is enough but for now I must decide what will be best to get me through the marathon, I don't want to affect the diet but I also don't want to get to twenty miles and be burnt out from the ketosis diet, I don't think I could cope with that.

CHAPTER SIX

MY FIRST MARATHON – DUBLIN 2011

The Dublin Marathon, and the immediate run up to it was one of the greatest experiences of my life. The real hype started a few days before it when Today FM's Jenny Kelly emailed me to see if I would go on RTÉ's *Saturday Night Show* with Ray, to talk about doing the marathon. I said yes, but only because Ray would be sitting beside me, other than that I think I'd have been too scared. It is a big show with a live audience – as far as you could get from the rest of my media experience to date.

A few days before the show I was contacted by Caroline, from *The Saturday Night Show*, and I went through my story with her. She also told me they were going to book Shelly and me into the Radisson St Helen Hotel, near RTÉ, on the Saturday night.

I was delighted when Chris asked me I'd like him to be with me on Saturday for the television stint. I had wanted to ask him if he could be there but hadn't liked to, since he is leaving his family for two nights as it was to do the marathon.

On the Thursday before the marathon, I couldn't go to college because of the radio interview, and, instead, went to my brother Darren's house, since we don't have a landline here. So, there I was, on air with Johnny Donnelly, and Gerry Duffy. Ray asked the three of us how we were feeling about Monday and if we had any game plans. I enjoyed the chat, and explained that, in relation to my game plane, which had been devised by Chris, our plan was to start at the front of the crowd, or as near to the front as we could get. That way people would pass us out, but it would take a while before the two of us would be left completely alone. If we started from the back we would be starting by ourselves from the very first step, since we were going to be walking and people tend to take off immediately at a ferocious pace. Mentally, this could prove to be potentially negative, and we wanted to make use of the atmosphere – the buzz – of walking within a crowd of fellow competitors, for as many miles as possible.

The two lads (Gerry Duffy and Johnny Donnelly) were very complimentary about me, and then Ray and I had a bit of banter about being on RTE this Saturday. I have to say though, that I much prefer being in the radio studio, it was a bit impersonal doing the interview by phone.

Afterwards I headed into town to pick up some bits and pieces for the weekend. I decided to buy myself a new pair of runners; a downside of my weight from a marathon perspective is that it simply compacts the runners very quickly so because my mileage is relatively high I need new runners every six to eight weeks and so I went into Limerick

Sports Store, where I buy all my stuff to get a new pair. Siobhan, the sales assistant, knew exactly what I was looking for and went off to the stockroom to get them. When she came back she told me that the manager, Christy, wanted a word with me. I couldn't believe it – Christy came out to me with the runners, worth €140, and handed them to me, as a gift, wishing me the best of luck on Monday from the shop. I didn't know what to say. Such generosity!

At this time, I had decided to come off the diet, but not to tell Motivation. Anyone I spoke to thought it was the wisest course of action. It just didn't seem healthy to walk for eight hours or so, on not much food and protein only, I really didn't want to compromise what I was doing as it wasn't all about a marathon more proving to myself I could do it and in some way hopefully discovering some new things about myself. I was sure the Motivation staff would understand, but I decided just to keep it to myself. It took me a while to make the decision and I didn't want to go into the ins and out of it.

The big day was getting closer and closer. On the Friday I swam and then headed into college, finishing up at 1pm. Jenny Kelly rang to wish me luck for the weekend. In the afternoon I had physio. Richard gave me a good rub down, followed by acupuncture on my feet and knees. They felt great after it. My foot, thank goodness, was a good bit better.

I had a small amount of porridge to see how my body reacted to it, it tasted strange, though maybe that was to do with the texture, and then I began to pack for Dublin.

On Saturday morning I had one last physio session this time with Emlyn Maher in TriFit, Emlyn spends the day in the gym helping all his customers selflessly; he should have been resting himself as he was also running on Monday, but the banter just added to the experience. After checking and re-checking my bags about ten times, at least, Shelly and I left for Dublin on Saturday at about 1pm. I wanted to stop off, on the way, at the shop, Mr Big Clothing, as I wasn't completely happy with the clothes I had picked for RTÉ. It is hard to know what to wear for something like this. Anyway, I was probably too distracted to concentrate on shopping and, after a few minutes, decided to stick with my own outfit.

We drove to the Radisson and checked in; both of us were completely overawed by the grandeur of the hotel, especially when we saw the suite that had been booked for us. Dinner was a small amount of pasta for me and then we both got ready. Chris arrived just before 8pm and we had an hour to chat before the chauffeured car arrived to pick the three of us up at 9pm. It was a very short trip, RTÉ is just down the road from the hotel, but it was long enough for me to start to feel exceedingly nervous.

On arrival at the studios we were shown to the Green Room, where some of the other guests, for the show, were chatting to one another. I don't know what I was expecting but it was quite small, around about the same size as a normal sitting-room, with some couches and chairs. At the side was a table covered in food, from crisps to assorted sandwiches. Naturally I didn't go near it. The room was full, though maybe there were only about twenty people in it, guests and their companions. None of them looked as nervous as I felt. Obviously nobody really knew who I was and I felt like the odd man out. Anyway I hadn't got time to feel too shy as one of the production assistants suddenly appeared to take me to have my make-up done. I followed her through reception just in time to meet Ray who arrived through the front door. He came with me to the make-up room which was a relief, I was glad to have him to talk to. On the way, we bumped into Brendan O'Connor, the show's presenter, who gave me a friendly welcome and asked was I nervous about the marathon. He also kindly told me that he knew what it was like to be on a diet, since he too had to watch his weight. I was relieved to have met him beforehand as his little chat did help to relax me a little.

In no time at all we were told it was time to go to the studio. Shelly and Chris were led to the audience while I followed Ray. As we stood behind stage, Ray kept me calm, telling me to just be myself, the way I was when I was in the Today FM studios, I must say it was a massive help to have Ray with me as I felt so relaxed. At home, Mam and Dad had their local switch on RTÉ so that they could watch me with some of their friends. They were so excited about the whole thing.

I went out first, and wasn't as terrified as I could have been. I mean, I knew the audience was sitting there, but really, the lights are so strong, and my heart was beating so loudly, I forgot to think about them, I couldn't really see them with the lights. Well, that's not exactly true. At some point, while I was telling my story, I suddenly became aware of all the people and it threw me off a little. I'm glad that I remembered to thank Ray and all his team for their help and support. Sure, I wouldn't have been sitting there if it wasn't for them.

Before I knew it, it was over. As I was leaving the stage someone shouted out, 'Good luck, Gary!' prompting more people to do the same. We made our way back to the Green Room. This time, when I walked in, everyone knew exactly who I was and congratulated me on the interview, which, in fairness, was nice. It was a wonderful experience. Little did I know that this support was just the start of it – and to think I had been a little uneasy about what people might think!

Ray headed off home shortly after that, while Chris drove back to Limerick. Shelly and I were chauffeured back to the hotel and headed for bed, after I replied to the many excited messages on my phone, from family and friends who had watched the show. I was too tired to do anything else. Now that the interview was out of the way my head is full of one thing and one thing only: Monday!

On Sunday 30 October, I woke up early, thanks to my excitement about the next day. We headed down to the restaurant for breakfast, which was nice; I had a little bit of everything: fruit, yoghurt, cereal and bread. Actually it was better than nice, it was heaven. It was a strange experience, eating 'real food', and really, hand on heart, what I enjoyed the most was the fruit. My tastebuds must have changed and been trained to appreciate the healthy stuff. The foods that I think I am going to faint over never prove to be as delicious as I expect them to be. I had a bit of a pastry, which was good, but I was able and happy enough to take just a couple of bites and put it back down again. These days, when I do break the diet, I love leaving food on my plate because the sight of uneaten food proves to me that I'm in control of my consumption and not the other way around. It was odd that some foods taste strange – milk for example isn't very nice as it tastes very sweet – I didn't need sugar in my tea and fruit really tasted good, almost as if I had never tasted it before.

I watched *The Saturday Night Show* on my laptop and was pleased with my performance. Nevertheless, I didn't really like when Brendan asked Ray if they only brought me onto the radio show so they could poke fun at me, and why didn't they just give me the scales. I wish now I had said something as without Ray and his team I don't think I would be on this amazing journey. Shelly went home, which was my choice. Selfish or not, I just wanted some space to myself today. I dropped her to the train and then checked into the Davenport where I had a nap before Chris arrived. He was late due to getting lost but eventually found our hotel at 5pm or so. We headed to the RDS (Royal Dublin Society) to register for the race, where we bumped into Chris' colleague, Emlyn, from Tri-Fit. Ray text me to go see Jim Aughney, the race director, to ask if he could help us start further up the front of the marathon crowd. Lots of people recognised me and wished me luck, which was both pleasant and overwhelming. Chris and I went to the Information Desk to ask about starting nearer the front and were given stickers to do just that. Because the attention we were receiving was a bit distracting, if well-meant, we left as soon as we sorted that out. While I really appreciate people's kind words I always feel awkward and never know what to say, as in my opinion, I am just doing what I need to do to get my life back. It may surprise people, but I never really understand why this has attracted so much attention or why people are so kind to me, but it is a massive encouragement for me.

Emlyn had invited us out to dinner with his friends so we both wanted to chill out at the hotel before that. At this stage nerves had well and truly set in, but I was just eager to get going. Our hotel was just beside the finish line so there was loads of activity around the hotel. We met up again and went to Milano, a restaurant just off the canal. It was a great way to spend the evening before a marathon. There were about

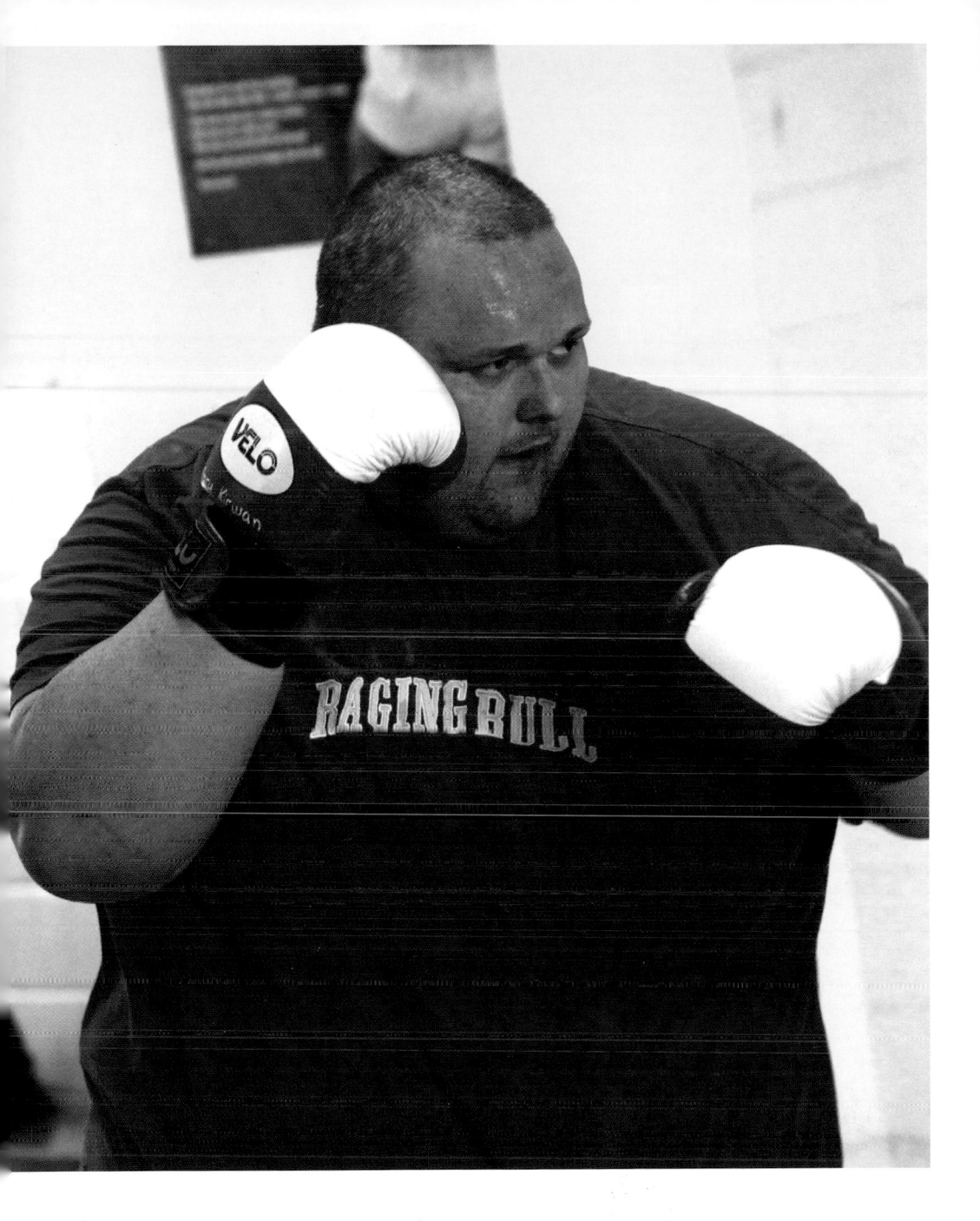

Above: Limerick Charity Boxing, May 2012; my first sporting challenge.

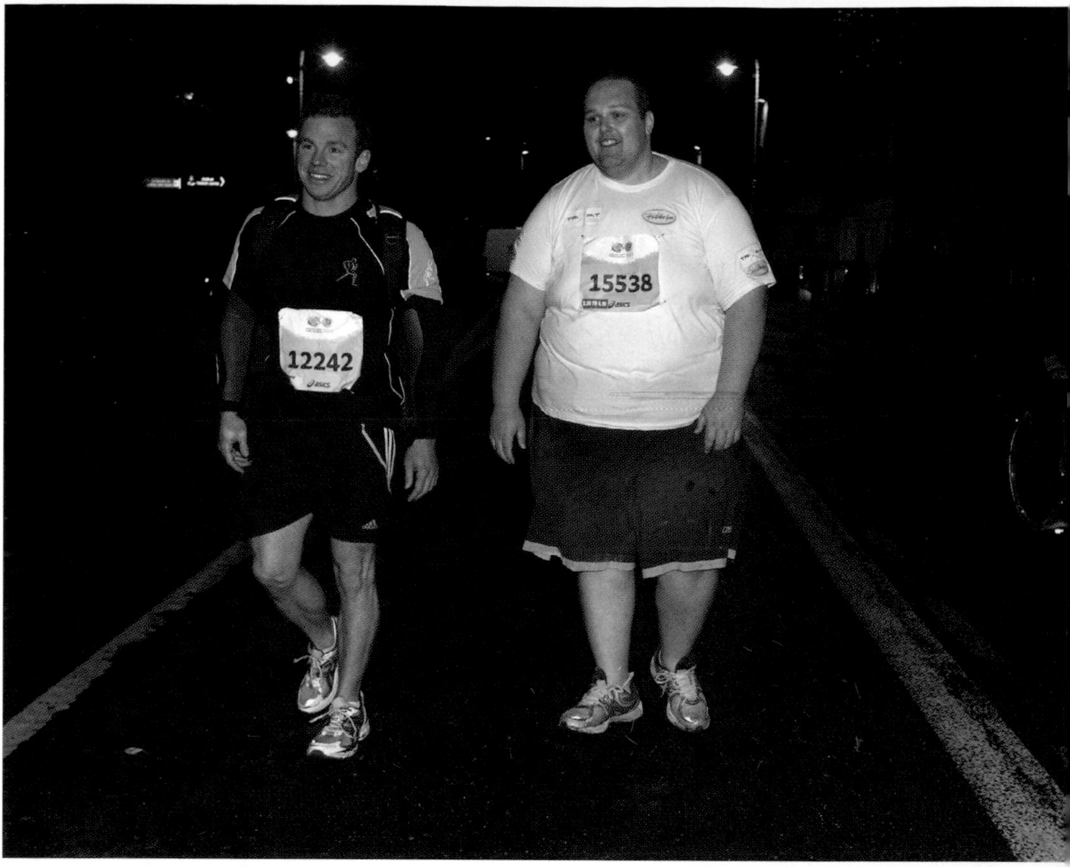
12242
15538

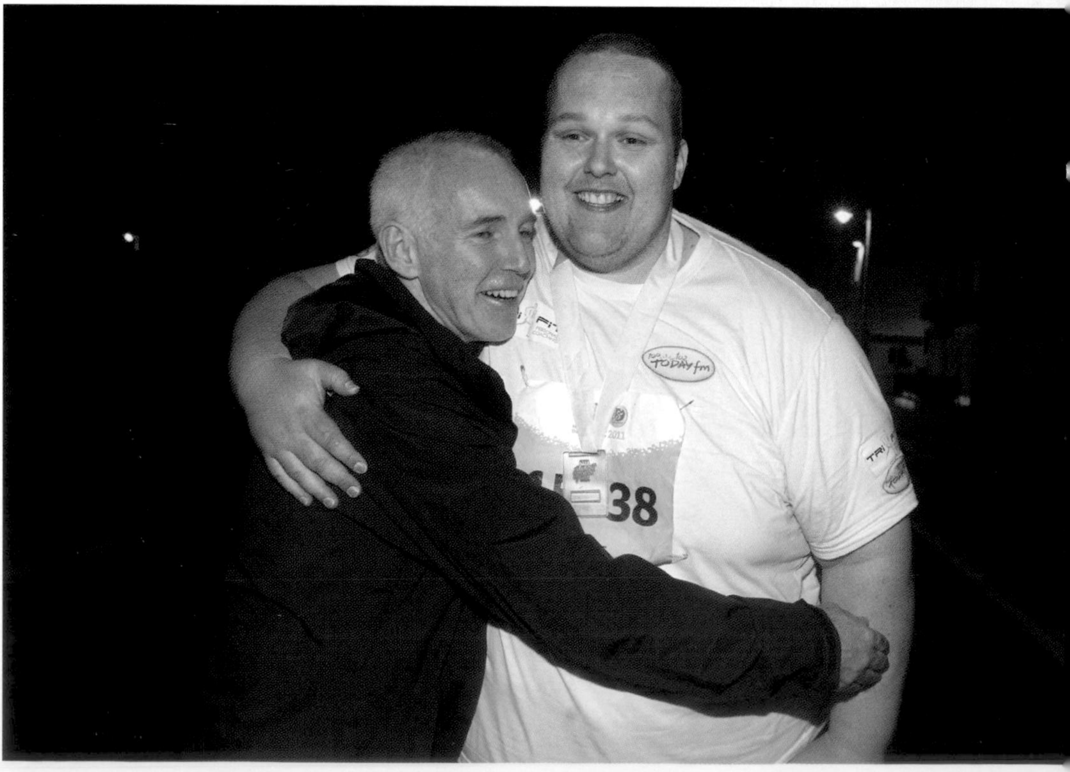
TODAY fm
38

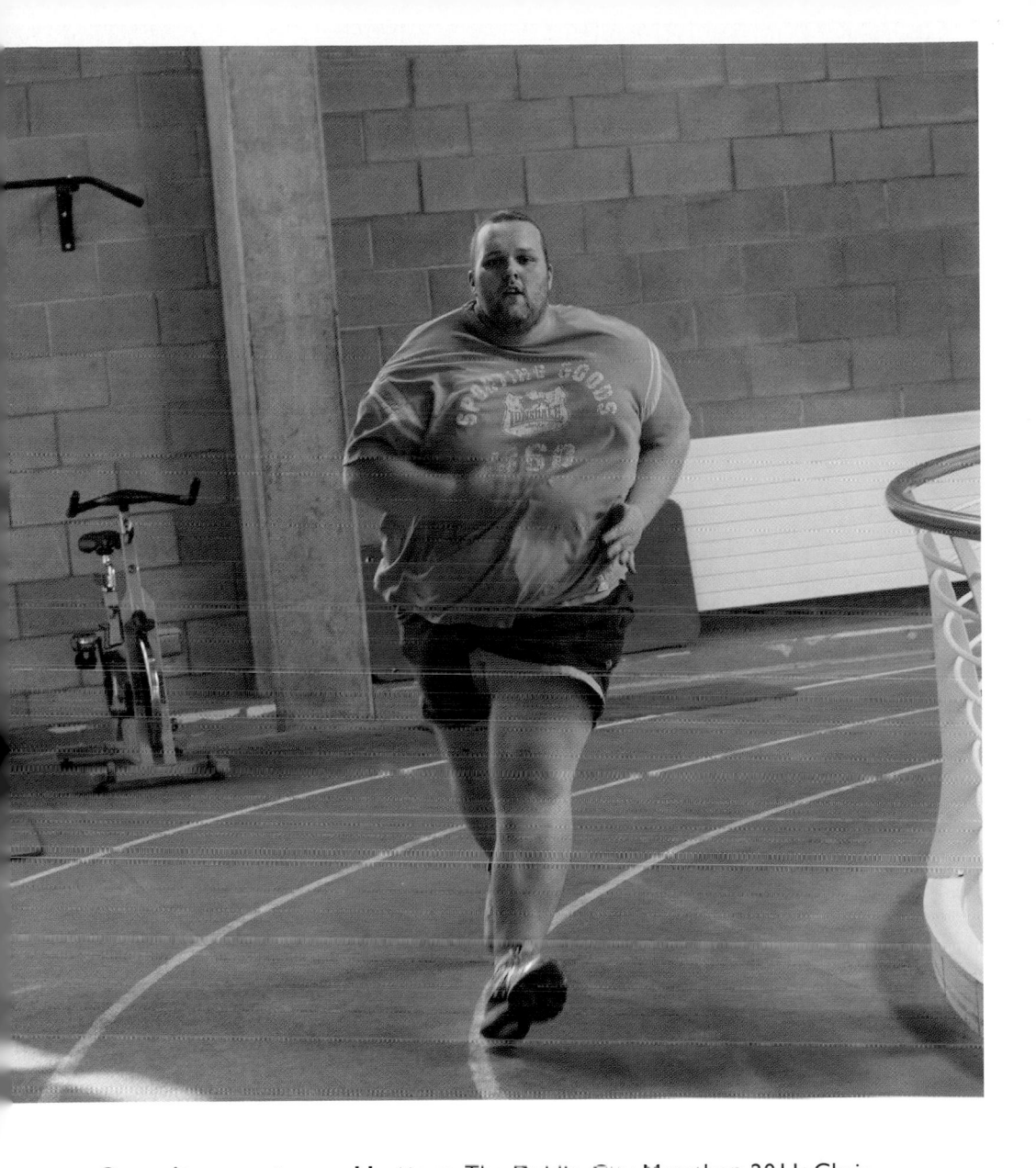

Opposite page, top and bottom: The Dublin City Marathon 2011: Chris and I smile wearily, but proudly, as we approach the finish line, and Ray D'Arcy congratulates me at the finish.

Above: On the indoor track in UL. I train as hard as I can and as often as I can. I love to run and am lucky that Limerick has such great facilities that I can use.

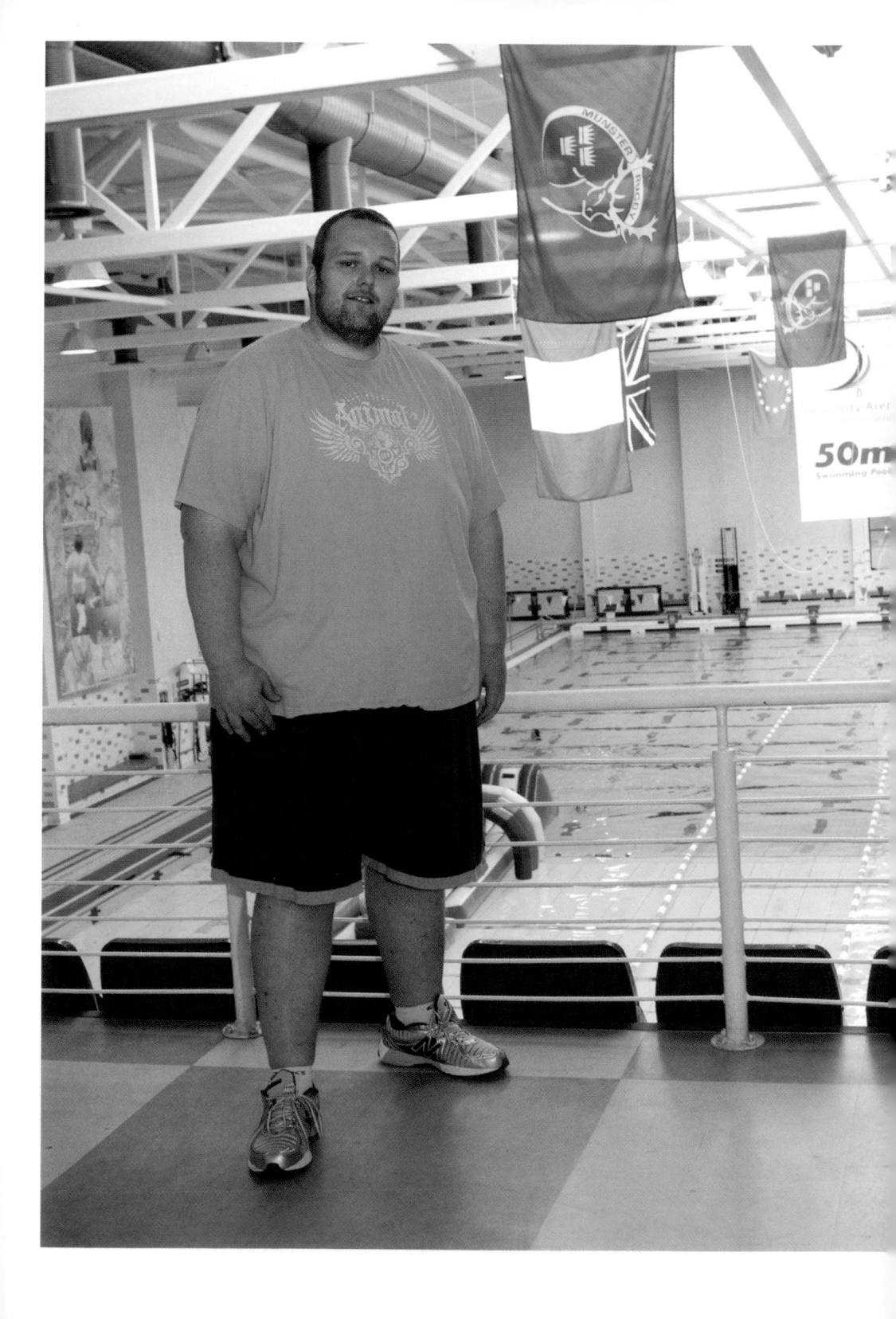

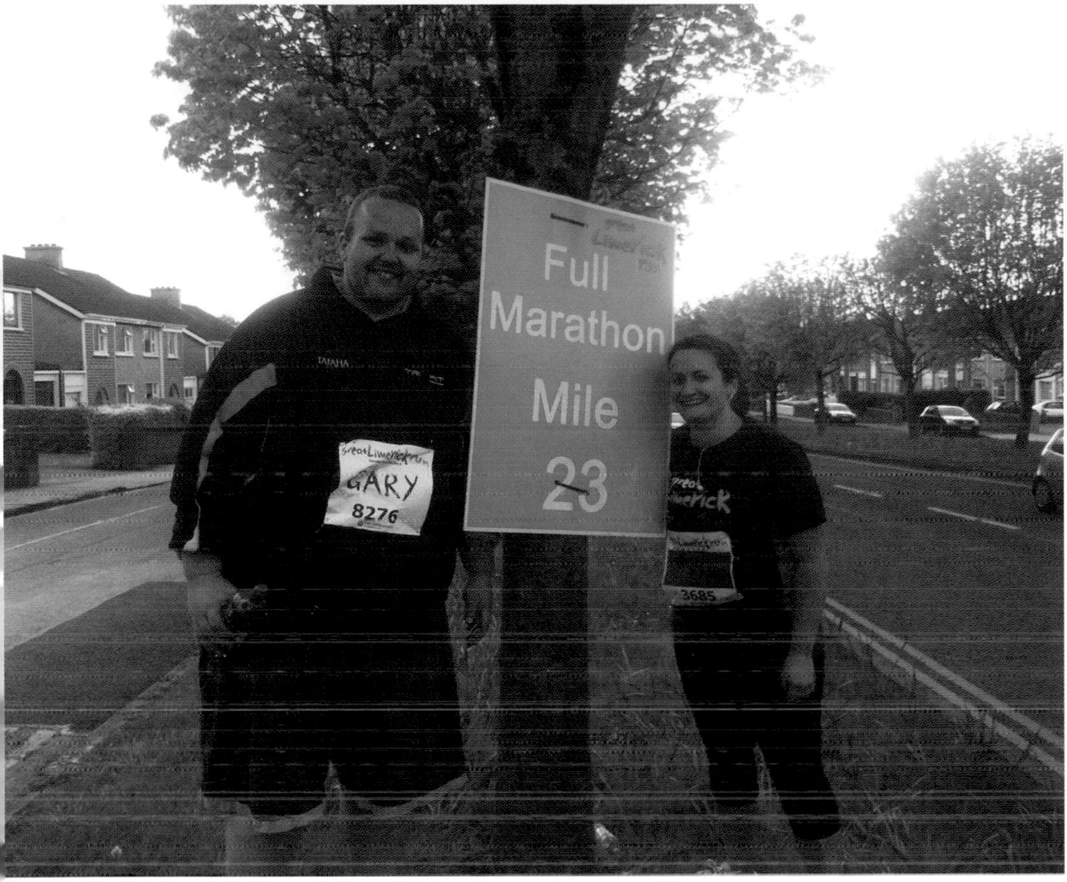

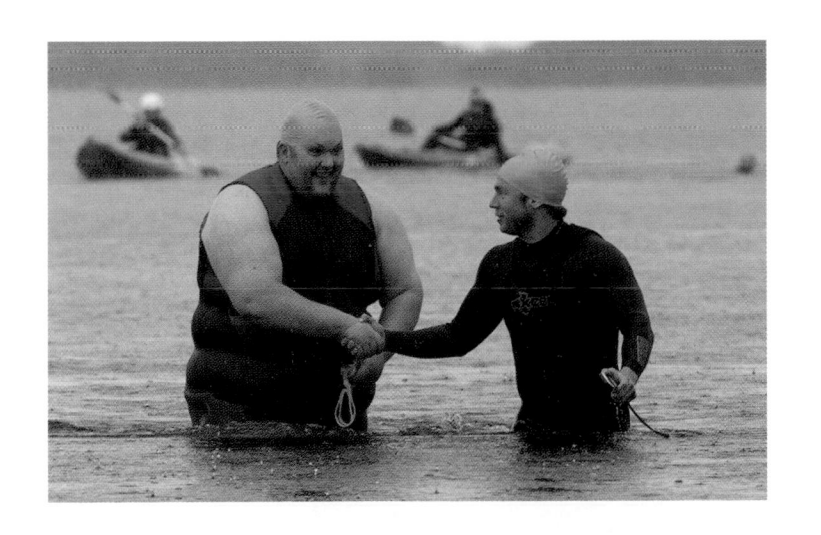

Opposite page: At the 50-metre pool in UL. Swimming has become so much a part of my life.

Above: With Denyse during the Great Limerick Run Marathon.

Below: A proud moment as Chris and I finish the i3 swim on a cold September morning, my first event where I didn't finish last.

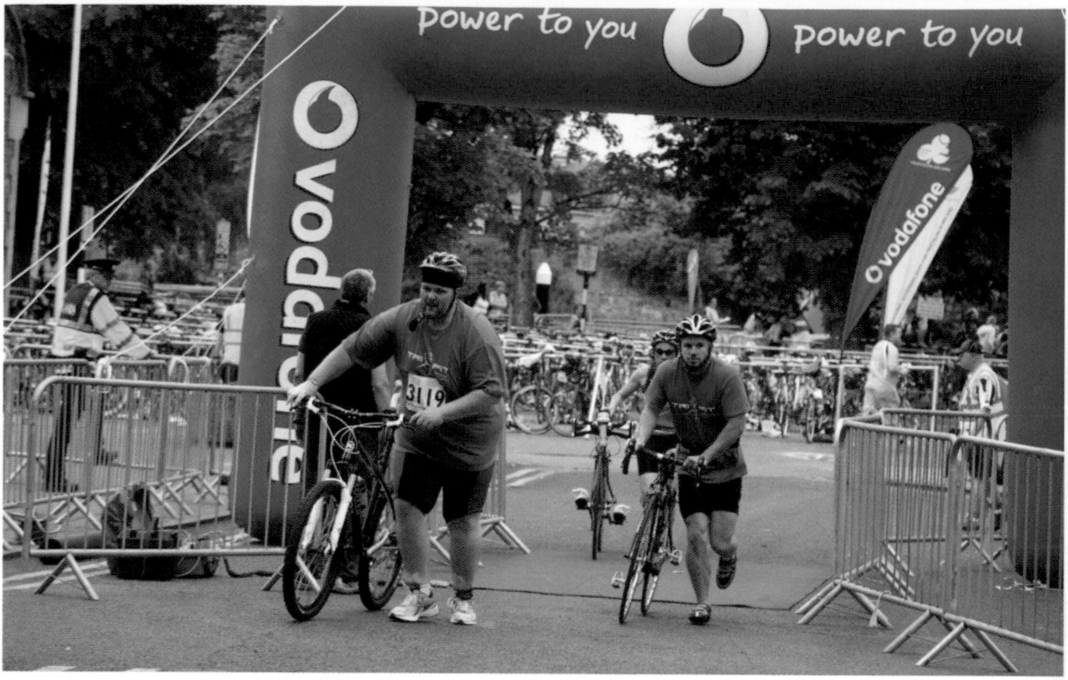
power to you
power to you
vodafone
vodafone
3119

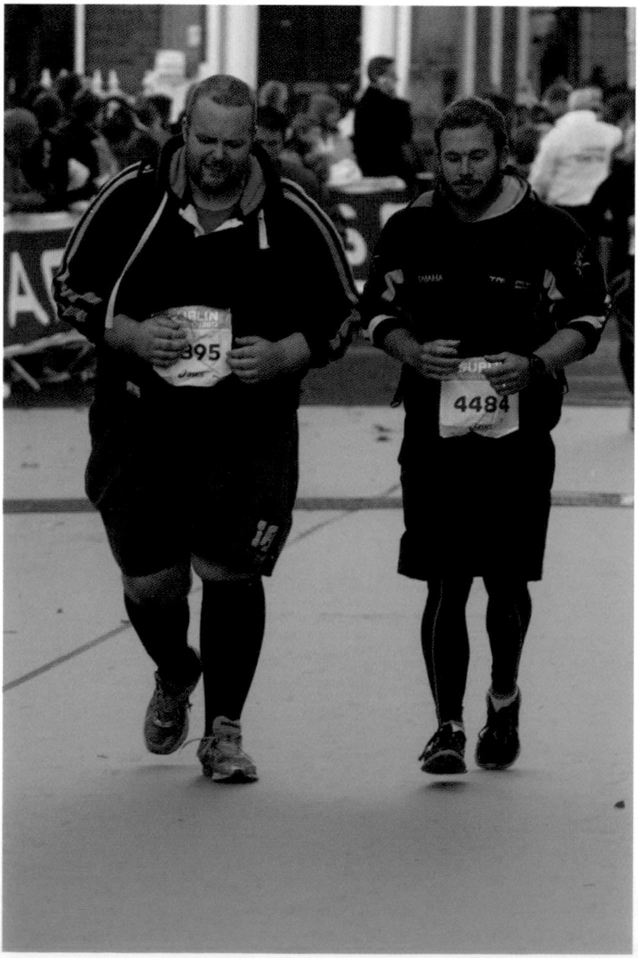
4484

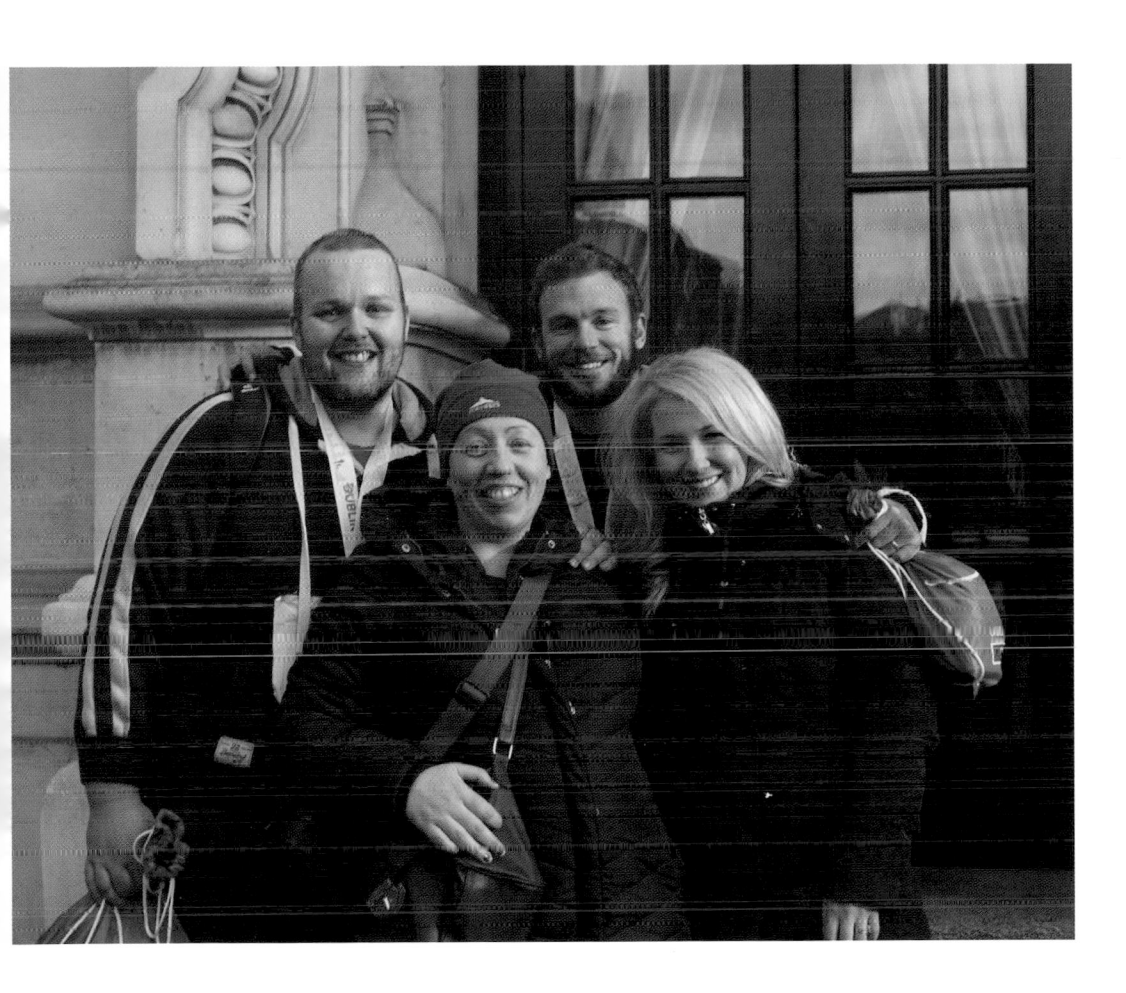

Opposite page top: Setting off on the cycle section at Try Athy. I hadn't been on a bike in ten years up until two days before this.

Opposite page bottom: Dublin City Marathon 2012: approaching the finish line, tired but triumphant with Chris.

Above: Chris and me with our beautiful wives, Shelly and Carly, after DCM 2012.

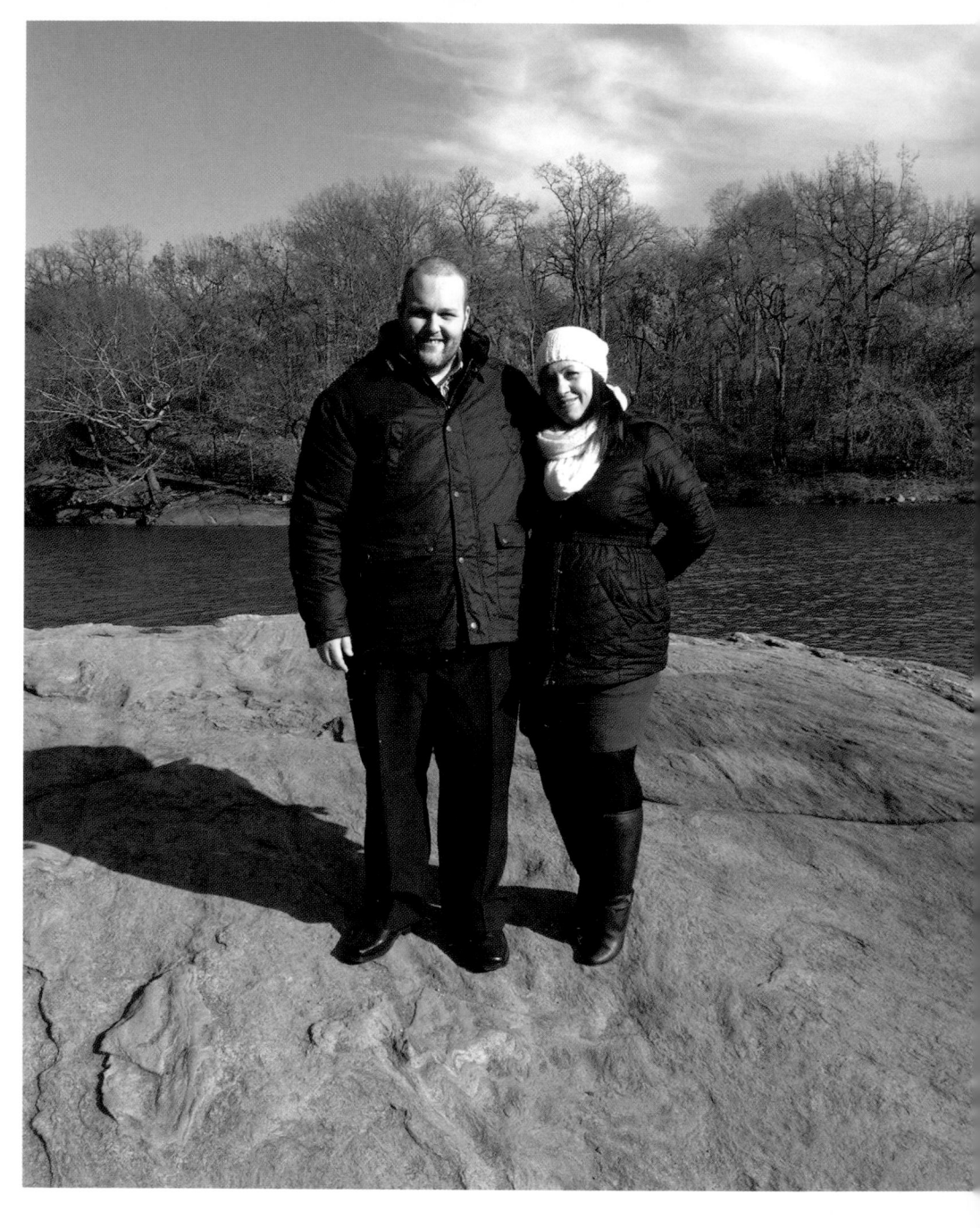

Above: Fit and happy on holidays in New York, 2012.

fourteen of us, some who had done the marathon before and some who were novices like me. It was exactly what I needed: good food, good company and good conversation. Chris had pizza while I ordered a dish of pasta and salad, but couldn't eat much of it because I was too nervous. Albeit, it was probably best not to finish it as I certainly didn't want to risk a bad stomach the night before the race.

Chris suggested getting a taxi back to the hotel but I was desperate to walk, having not done much walking in the last couple of days. We got a good look at the start/finish line, I wanted to take a picture of me under the finish line as I knew I wouldn't see it the following day, but Chris wouldn't allow me, he said he wanted me to wait until we cross the line tomorrow for that pic when we had earned it. I could not believe I was doing the marathon the next day. For the first time, in a long time, I really, really felt like I belonged to something big, special and inspiring. This was something I hadn't expected to feel, and it was bloody wonderful.

MONDAY, 31 OCTOBER: THE DUBLIN MARATHON!

I was wide awake at 6.30am, and absolutely raring to go. I couldn't believe the day was finally here and I can only compare it to the feeling I used to get as a child on Christmas morning. Chris and I had planned on a 7.30am breakfast, but he also woke up early so we headed downstairs at 7.00am. The restaurant had a unique atmosphere – excitement and nervousness mixed together almost like we were going to war. Still we both managed to relax a bit over the meal, and enjoy sitting there. We were very good, eating small portions of porridge, fruit and yoghurt, to be honest with nerves I did well to eat even that small amount of food.

After we had eaten we went outside to walk around the general area of the finish line. With two hours still to go until the start of the race, I knew I couldn't have handled sitting quietly in the hotel room. In fact there were quite a few people hanging around, doing the same thing.

When we were ready, we headed back to the room, stuck on loud music and took our showers. We started to get ourselves ready, me taking extra care to prepare my feet for the day ahead. Chris's Dad rang from Sydney to wish us luck, teasing Chris over the fact he had always said he would never do a marathon.

Chris started our warm up with some stretches and he got me to focus on what was ahead, what it meant to me and why I was here. I suppose from Chris's previous experience in sports, including playing for Munster he knew how to channel my nervous energy and get me ready for what lay ahead.

I made a few nervous trips to the bathroom and couldn't wait to get out of the hotel again. Chris filled his backpack with supplies for the both of us, including extra runners, talc powder, food and other bits and pieces. I handed Chris €20 in case we had forgotten anything. We took time to do stretching exercises and, at last, it was 9am and time to go outside.

The hotel lobby was full of people, including Gerry Duffy, who kindly took the time to talk to me and give me the simplest of advice. He spoke about belief, and that I might reach a stage later on when I stop believing that I can do this. 'When this happens,' he told me, 'break it down, all the way down, to one more step, one more step, one more step, and keep doing that because, before you know it, you will be a few hundred metres down the road and then you will be a mile, and you'll be over the worse part.' It was a privilege to have the opportunity to speak with such an accomplished athlete as Gerry before the marathon.

The three of us headed outside where we met Jonny and Ray, and then the five of us posed for photographs. I was recognised by Jane McKenna, who set up the LauraLynn Foundation, after losing her two daughters, Laura and Lynn, within two years of one another. She introduced herself to me, telling me how she found my story to be hugely inspiring. I could feel tears welling up in my eyes but, fortunately, managed to prevent them from spilling over. This woman has been to hell and back, and here she is telling me that I am inspiring. I have never felt so humbled and totally inadequate as having such an amazing person praise me.

So many people have their different reasons for doing this race, it makes for an emotionally-charged atmosphere, and it is humbling to be part of it. I did my best not to think too much about myself, and about the journey I had taken to get to stand here, I just wanted to savour this atmosphere. This time last year I probably spent the entire day on the couch, believing I had no future, no reason to get up in the morning, unable to do basic housework, unable to share a bed with my wife, afraid to leave the safety of my home.

Unsure about whether I was going to cry or not, I followed Chris to the starting area, in a daze. As we walked through the crowd I was aware that not one single person looked at me like I shouldn't be there. I think this is the beauty of marathons; there are so many people, of different shapes and sizes, of all ages, that nobody sticks out anymore than anyone else. In other words, we all fit in! It really is the most amazing feeling; here I was thirty stone at a marathon and I felt like I belonged there.

Since we were part of the second wave of runners, Chris and I had to wait down an alley before heading out to Fitzwilliam Street. I lost count of the amount of people who shook my hand and wished me well. I felt like I was about to walk onto a massive stage, such was the sense of expectation and excitement all around me – albeit this special feeling was only slightly marred by the smell of urine in the alley, due to umpteen people taking the opportunity to make pit stops before the race began.

Just before it was time to head out I took off my jumper. A special moment for me, I suppose, that nobody would have known about. There I was in a crowd of runners, taking off my jumper, with no shame or guilt. All those years when I wore the biggest jumpers Mam could find for me, hoping to hide my body from the sneers and countless unfunny jokes.

The National Anthem was played and it was time for our crowd to shuffle out from the dark alley into the blazing daylight on Fitzwilliam Street. And we were off! My natural instinct was to break into a run, just because I was so keyed up, but Chris had foreseen this and warned me, 'Whatever you do, don't start running, mate. We have a long day ahead of us, so let's take it slow and steady'. Then I scared the life out of the both of us by tripping over a can that had been thrown on the ground – I went over on my ankle and stumbled. Chris stared at me in horror until I gasped, 'I'm okay!'

We started off in the middle of 'Wave Two' but when we reached St Stephen's Green we looked back and saw 'Wave Three' coming at us, which was pretty special. For that first mile all I could hear and see were people wishing me well, shouting my name and clapping me on the back as they overtook me. As we came around by Trinity College an old man of maybe eighty years or so, jogged calmly passed us, impressing me and Chris no end. We headed onto O'Connell Street, where the crowd started to thin out a bit, allowing me to find a comfortable pace and get myself sorted mentally for the challenge. Unlike most of the other competitors, who would be going home in a few hours, I knew that I had eight hours plus of walking to go. Also, judging by the sky, we were going to be in for some rain, but I didn't mind the rain, as long as there was no wind. Chris and I continued to motor on nicely, not feeling the need to chat unless there was something to say.

There was a shitty moment as we hit Dorset Street. A couple of druggies spotted me in the crowd and began to loudly chant, in between peals of nasty laughter, 'You're last! You're last!' It didn't bother me in the least. I merely shot them – what I hope was – a look of utter smugness, thinking, '*I don't see you gobshites doing this!*' Chris, however, had a different reaction, as in a more pro-active one, and I had to stop him from marching right over to them. I think he was taken aback by how cruel these taunts were and I knew by his reaction he would have had more than a friendly word!

We continued on and grinned bravely when even Santa passed us by, until, suddenly, it seemed that we were alone. People had stopped overtaking us as we went hit the third mile and the first water station. It was a little disheartening, I had been sure we would be surrounded by people for ages yet. We approached the Phoenix Park at a good, strong pace and had a bite to eat from Chris' backpack. Regarding food, the plan was to keep our intake little and often. Our mood was still a little heavy from the episode with the junkies. Chris turned to me and said, 'No matter how tough it gets today, just keep putting one foot in front of the other and we'll get to the finish line'. I nodded and assured him, 'No matter how painful it gets today, it can never match the pain I used to have when people looked at me in disgust. If I keep remembering that, nothing will stop me from crossing that finish line!' The relief on Chris' face was enormous; he really wanted us to do this together, until the very end. I think it was one of those rare moment when two men share their feelings openly and honestly. I wasn't trying to be profound, but this is what I had used to motivate me in the past few weeks and while at times it was painful to relive some of those looks and words I also knew that today would in some ways allow me to break free of those memories and move far beyond them.

As we reached the park a St John's ambulance began to trail us, for which I was far from grateful, but, after a while, was able to ignore it. We happened upon a group of six adults and ten kids. As soon as the kids spotted us they ran for us cheering, 'Gary! Gary! Gary!' I have to say they made my day. They and their parents had stood and waited especially for us so that they could lend their support. It completely made up for earlier, and then some, I think this is probably one of the highlights of the last two years and probably something I will always remember with a big smile on my face. The Phoenix Park was also a particularly nice part of the route; it was so quiet and peaceful. It was my first time to see it like this; I had only ever visited the zoo there. I knew that when we came out the other side we would have walked eight miles, a third of the way. Just as I had with the diet, from the very beginning, when facing into the amount of weight I had to lose, I broke the race up into a series of smaller, more manageable goals.

As I began to feel that everything was going perfectly, out of the blue both my calves and Achilles tendons tightened which shocked me and was a little disheartening. Even on the longest walks I had performed, in training for today, this had never happened, and for it to be happening so early in the race was a bit of a bombshell. We had to stop to allow me to stretch my legs. It seemed to work, the muscles loosened, and we continued on again for a few steps, but then the muscles painfully tightened again. So we would walk until I had to stop, and stretch the muscles until I could continue walking again, which was something neither of us had catered for when we were making out our time-schedule for the race.

By mile six, and water station two, we had just accepted our bottles of water when the roads in the park were re-opened, sending us both swiftly to the paths, as traffic flowed once more. But the paths were awkward to keep to so we returned to the roads, in between the passing traffic, which brought us to the attention of the Park Rangers, who requested that we get back on the paths. Fortunately, the staff in the St John's ambulance came to our aid. They trailed us, in the ambulance, providing a barrier between us and the cars. We stayed on the road and didn't have to worry about being hit, and I was immensely grateful to them this time.

By the time we reached the end of the Phoenix Park, any dreams we were holding of a seven-hour walk were well and truly gone. I started to realise we could still have eight or nine hours ahead of us, at the rate we were going, thanks to my legs. We reached the last water station standing, there would be no more water handed to us after this point, which was a hindrance, as it meant that Chris now had to carry a lot of extra water in the backpack. Normal traffic resumed everywhere so we really had to stick to the paths now and it was a bit lonely since we were the only competitors around. I knew this would happen, but I didn't think it would happy so early on in the day, which really brought me down from the amazing high of the start line just two hours ago.

Just as my head started to droop we came down the Chapelizod Road to find a couple waiting for us. They knew the drink stations were gone and so stood with bottles of Lucozade, determined that we would have something to drink. They were like an oasis in the desert, except that they were real. I couldn't thank them enough for their kindness and consideration.

After we left them things got a bit glum. We plodded along and had to search for signs that we were still on the race track, until, that is, our saviours, the St John's ambulance, arrived once more. They drove ahead and then pulled in until we passed by, and then would drive on another bit to wait for us before letting us walk by again. It was like a game of leapfrog, but they helped us stay confident that we were, at least, on the right road.

Just as we started into the ninth mile, the heavens opened. It was tough but – silver linings and all that – it did distract me from the pain in my legs. I glanced at Chris and said, 'At least it won't be bloody raining in the desert!' The rain lasted for ages, and my body temperature started to drop from being wet, making me cramp even worse. Chris rang Carly, his wife, who was with Shelly, and asked them to bring Deep Heat and Voltarol, which we hoped would help with my cramps. We were unsure as to exactly where we were, though we knew we were somewhere on the Crumlin Road. The girls got a taxi and made him drive the length of the road until they found us. By this stage I was in a bad way, and although I knew I wasn't going to give up no matter what, it seemed to me that my body was letting me down and, therefore, I was losing confidence in myself; to be perfectly honest I was in physical and mental hell. Because of all this, I didn't want to face Shelly and let her see how miserable I was. So I did something shitty. I let Chris take the stuff from the taxi while I briefly smiled in at my wife and kept walking, a very hard thing to do, but I knew if I stopped I would fall apart. The clean-up crews arrived to clean up after the race, which did not help to lift our spirits in the least, plus our ambulance had gone missing so we had to worry about not going off course and ending up God knows where.

The rain finally stopped four miles later, marking the half-way point. This was a bit of a mile stone alright. Also we were going to be walking downwards for the rest for the next while. Thanks to all this I began to feel a pull towards positivity for the first time since we entered the Phoenix Park. We still had to stop frequently and let me stretch my leg muscles, but our pace had quickened as our mood brightened a little; at least it had stopped raining. We reached 13.5 miles and the ambulance re-joined us, stopping to ask if we would like a lift some of the way. Now, I know the man was just being kind but, Jesus Christ, I was really pissed off. There was no way I was going to stop walking the race, no matter what time it was or where we were, and by doing this, completing the course, I was making a statement. I was showing the world I was not a piece of shit and, in my own way, was responding to every single dirty look I had ever received in my entire life. I'm sure

I came across as being ungracious but I was too knackered to worry about it.

About a half mile later we were joined by Lorraine Turner, one of Chris' colleagues from TriFit, and her friend, who arrived on their bikes, from which they promptly dismounted in order to walk with us for a while. This was a huge help since what we badly needed were distractions from pain, tiredness and the distance we still had to cover. As we walked together a man came running out of his house to ask Chris and me if we needed anything. This was another welcome boost, because he reminded us that we were part of something and not two lonely, damp men doing some sort of Forrest Gump in the middle of nowhere.

At mile sixteen we said goodbye to the girls and they were replaced by new visitors, in the form of Gerry Duffy, his girlfriend and his sister. They had driven along the route looking for us to make sure we were okay. On seeing us, they pulled over, got out of the car and began to walk with us, keeping our spirits up with chat and support. As we walked along I thought I was imagining things when I saw some people, in the distance, who sort of looked like my parents and god-daughter, Nicole. It was them! They had decided to surprise me and this they certainly achieved. I was so glad to see them, but could do no more than hug them quickly and keep moving; believing that if I stood still for even a second my body would give up and I wouldn't be able to move again. They walked with us for a few minutes before wishing me luck for the rest of the race. For some reason I thought my heart would break as they left. I just felt really sad to see them go. Gerry and the others left soon after but not before he made sure we had plenty of food and water to keep us going. Both my family and Gerry had given me a huge mental boost. I know I didn't really show my appreciation, but it did if only for a few minutes, take me out of hell.

It was just Chris and I once more, and the going got hard as most of the signs, showing the way, had been removed, plus it was starting to get dark. I must admit, it was more than a bit depressing. Miles eighteen and nineteen were difficult in that we were unsure if we were still on the route. At one stage I thought Chris said we needed to cross the main road and took off across the busy road to find I was alone. I looked back for Chris and he was standing on the path I had just left, gazing after me in total disbelief and misery. Realising my mistake I crossed back over and burst out laughing at Chris' face. I was wrecked, wet and freezing cold, what else was there to do but laugh.

Mile nineteen was the last time we would find any evidence of road signs pointing the way forward. I suppose it is a credit to the efficiency of the clean-up crews, they had certainly done their jobs well, while also making it difficult for us to find our bearings. Thankfully we hailed a passing cyclist who told us where we were and where we were going. He also gave us a wonderful boost when he told us that there were other competitors not too far ahead. Thank God! We weren't the only ones still going through hell! Knowing there were others still on the course made me feel like I was not quite alone; it's pretty strange the things you grasp on to when in such pain!

Just approaching mile twenty we met a girl called Angela, who was on her way to her local shop. When she saw us she stopped in her tracks with a look of utter surprise, a very different look to what I was used to and asked if I was the guy from the *Saturday Night Show*, and when

I said 'yes', asked if she could walk with us for a bit. She was a blessing because she was so friendly and chatty and, by now, we would have talked to anyone to escape however briefly the mental and physical torture of those remaining miles. We breezed through the next half mile, thanks to Angela, and she gave us solid directions for the next bit of the journey, before saying goodbye and before we really hit the wall.

Just after Angela came Heartbreak Hill, it was dark we were wet and very cold, there were no signs on the course. We looked like the walking dead and I felt like it also. Not only had I hit the wall, I felt like the wall had fallen on me.

When we finally reached UCD (University College Dublin, Belfield) I had a vague idea of the area, which was a comfort, but this is when things began to slow right down to a snail's pace for me, I was at that stage that Gerry Duffy had described, but much worse I was struggling to even make one or two steps at a time. We had now been walking for seven or eight hours and the end was still quite a bit away yet. It is hard to say which was worse, the mental or the physical battle. At mile twenty-one we headed down Fosters Avenue and onto the Stillorgan Road, where most runners hit a wall and I can well believe it. It's the worst part of the course, mostly because it's such a busy road. Also it is pretty difficult to tell how far you are from the city, and not to have a decent idea regarding the distance in front of us played havoc with my motivation and emotions, I was really down at this point. Nevertheless we met another lovely guy who hung around to give us, and any other stragglers, water and food. I thought it was the most wonderful thing to do, to be out there, hours and hours later, to make sure anyone who was still in the race was okay for supplies. We walked towards the flyover, on the Stillorgan Road, to cross over by RTÉ when a car pulled up beside us, I initially took no notice until I heard our names being called and out popped Ray D'Arcy. He and Jenny had been ringing to see how I was and when they couldn't get through to me, due to the O2 network being down, Ray came out looking for us. It was brilliant to see him. He gave us directions and offered us clothes. Okay, so nothing he had would go near me but he pushed Chris who said no, which made no sense at all since we were walking in damp, smelly clothes. I don't think either of us was able to think properly, we were just on auto-pilot.

Ray drove back home and we continued on for RTÉ, on the lookout for a shopping centre that Ray told us would be nearby. Unfortunately he had also said we needed to take a right at RTÉ. What is unfortunate about that is, instead of turning right, we walked on past the building. I don't know how far we went before we realised that there was no sign of a shopping centre, then we were suddenly at Donnybrook Stadium, which I knew we definitely were not supposed to pass and we knew we were in trouble and rang Ray to discover we were lost. I was hanging on by a thread at this point and to hear that we had walked extra on top of what we still needed to do was … actually, I don't think I have the words to describe just how utterly horrible that was. We managed to get back on track and find our way to Ballsbridge, where a guy, who was smoking outside a pub, put us right and delivered the most fantastic news: the finish line was just two miles away. The strange thing was while it was great news and lifted me mentally, physically I was still telling myself 'one more step'. I was still stopping every fifteen minutes or so to stretch as I was seizing up at this stage; never in my life had two miles felt so far away.

We headed down the Shelbourne Road, coming up against a bunch of young girls who looked like they were on the way to a disco. As we passed them one of them exclaimed, 'You're the guy from TV!' When I confirmed that I was he, they started high-fiving us which, at this stage in the proceedings, gave us both the giggles while dutifully high-fiving them back. We left them slowly, mainly because our pace was down to a crawl, but it was a pleasantly-surreal event that made us both laugh. I was a bit worried about my body remaining functional for the last couple of miles but, in fairness, I really didn't have the energy to worry that much about it. We were now living purely in the moment, from step to step.

Just before we crossed the Grand Canal, we passed by a pub near the Aviva Stadium and heard a shout from inside, 'Go on, Gary, you're nearly there!' God himself couldn't have sounded sweeter at that point. On we went, crossing a bridge over the Grand Canal when a car pulled up beside us, flashing its lights, and someone was cheering for us. It took me a few seconds to understand it was Ray again, with Jenny and their daughter. They decided to come out to be with us to ensure we didn't get lost again. I try hard to explain to people just how supportive these two have always been and now here they were, having dragged their daughter out into a cold, damp evening to make sure that Chris and I knew where we were going and that we were OK. It was above and beyond the call of duty and went far beyond the requirements of the radio show.

Ray did exactly what we needed him to do, he chatted away, keeping us occupied so that we might forget just how exhausted we were. I began to feel I was having a surreal, or even a sort of supernatural experience, as we headed into the last mile. There I was, with Chris and Ray, two men who had done so much in helping me transform my life. It is something that I will never forget. At that point I began thinking about someone else who had been there for me, all the way through, Shelly. Chris and I had been trying to call the girls, not realising that the O2 network was down temporarily. Finally we reached them and told them we were nearly there. Ray cleared his throat and told us that there was still a lap to be done around Trinity College. From the sound of his voice I knew he dreaded having to tell us this but no matter, whatever was left to do we were going to finish this race properly.

On Fenian Street we passed the Davenport's car-park. I am sure that Chris will agree with me that there has never been a more emotional sighting of a car-park in the whole, wide world. We came around by the hotel and had to veer right for the last lap. A photographer joined us, which was another good distraction. My cramp disappeared as we strolled up by Trinity College in fact it had stopped after Ray joined us as he offered such a massive distraction. We headed towards Clare Street and I took off my damp jumper. It was the strangest feeling; there, just in front, was the finishing line! Well actually there was no line, but I knew where it should be from the night before so I knew this was the last few hundred metres. All day I was in hell and after over ten and a half hours, for the first time I knew I was going to finish! It was so surreal as I had spent the day knowing I could do it, but to switch from 'I will' to 'I am' was a crazy feeling As we approached the finish I was very surprised as there were quite a few people standing around it. Instinctively I straightened my posture, like a cyclist coming to the end of the Tour de France. I gathered myself.

Ray quietly disappeared off to the side, leaving Chris and me as we had started out this morning, walking side by side, just the two of us. To be honest I would have liked Ray to stay with us. As we crossed the junction with just thirty metres to go we could finally see the faces in the crowd, we could see the our wives who marking the line and we headed to them; I just wanted to hold Shelly.

As we came to a stop and the journalists fired questions at me. Shelly grabbed me by the hand and pulled me over the line, pointing it out to me. It was so surreal, but to be honest I don't know how I didn't collapse. While I was so happy to finish I just wanted to sit down – but not before getting my medal and a few pictures.

What a day it was. It was such proof in the improvement in my confidence that I stood in a crowd of fifteen thousand runners and did not feel out of place. One of my favourite moments had to be those kids, in the Phoenix Park, who were cheering for me and chanting my name. However, the whole experience was made more wonderful by the fact that I got to share that entire torturous day with my trainer. He was – quite literally – there for me, every little step of the way and throughout it all he kept me smiling even when I was in hell.

We all had beer and pizza the night of the marathon and I had no qualms at all about consuming either of them! The amount of texts, phone calls and hugs I got, on crossing that line was unreal. Gerry Duffy had sent a friend to wait for us. There were two soldiers who had finished before us and who had carried full packs on their marathon; they waited around to see us finish which meant a lot to me. Ray D'Arcy was hugging and beaming at us like a proud parent. The girls were relieved it was over; Shelly had been worried all day about me and understandably so since, for the most part, they had no idea where we were. And the amount of photographers and journalists who surrounded us made me feel like some sort of movie star.

Shelly found out our official time: we had walked for ten hours and forty-six minutes.

I was in bed by midnight, just three hours after finishing the race. The relief in lying down on that mattress was immense, and I was absolutely primed to go unconscious as soon as I shut my eyes. Therefore, it was bewildering when, a little while later, to feel my body going into agony instead of the ecstasy of sleep. I was awake until 2.30am or so, in pain, with the biggest smile on my face.

It was equally shocking to be wide awake at 7am the next morning, but I was dying to get to Today FM and talk about the whole experience, I really just wanted to thank all those who had helped me the day before as what they did got me through the day even though they probably will never realise the importance of what they did. I tended to my blistered feet, showered, dressed and headed down for breakfast where I was soon joined by Chris. We were both on a high from the marathon. The girls joined us; Shelly had run out to get some newspapers in which we featured and we poured over them in delight. Then we had the most truly divine breakfast, not that I ate much, but I allowed myself a pick at everything: fruit, bread and cereal, before getting ready for Today FM.

The interview was a thrilling blur. I did my best to mention everyone I had met and who had helped us out, while also trying to describe as much as I could, in fifteen minutes. I just wanted to be able to share the experience with Ray and his team because so much was down to their support. Texts of congratulations flooded in from the listeners and everyone in the studio was so excited for us. I could have stayed there for hours on end but, of course, we had to leave and return to the world outside.

Back at the hotel we all packed up, checked out and then Shelly and I said goodbye to Carly and Chris, who were staying around Dublin for the rest of the day. We got in our car and headed back to Limerick, getting home around 1pm, just before I crashed.

My body went into shock. I lay on the couch for a few hours, shaking and in pain, before giving in and going to bed, stumbling up the stairs like a drunken person. The whole family came to visit me, but I was hardly aware of them being there.

Even at this stage the enormity of what I had done hadn't quite sunk in, but what had sunk in and what was such a huge surprise to me was how kind people were; while I used to fear a certain look I had experienced a new look one that for me allowed me to break free off my past and move on with my life.

Wednesday, 2 November:

Wow, am I stiff and sore today but, thank God, I'm nowhere near as bad as I was last night. That was freaky! I guess my body just hit a wall and continued to hit it for hours on end. Shelly went to college and I went to UL for the most gorgeous swim. It was pure luxury, stretching out my limbs in the water and not feeling any pain.

I could take time to think about my achievement: **I, Gary Kirwan, completed the Dublin City marathon**. Who would have believed it! Yet, while I am so pleased of that particular accomplishment, I can't help but remind myself that doing the marathon has nothing much to do with the diet, and I'm only half-way through that race.

My poor feet are going to be wrapped up for a week, they are in a bit of state but that was only to be expected.

Friday, 4 November:

My body is slowly returning to normality, though I am still quite sore in my hips, ass and knees.

Chris had me do a light session in the gym tonight, just to go through the motions.

Monday, 7 November: (Week 11)

I trained tonight but am not feeling great. My throat is sore and I think I am coming down with another chest infection.

Tuesday, 8 November:

When I woke up this morning, I felt I had a hangover. Don't feel good at all.

Wednesday, 9 November:

I went into college but was forced to leave after just one lecture, and drive straight to the doctor with a list of complaints: kidney infection, chest infection, and temperature, to name but a few. He told me it was all a result of what I put my body through on Monday, ordering me to rest for a few days and giving me a prescription for antibiotics.

Even though I'm freezing, as I sit here typing this, the sweat is pouring out of me. I cannot remember when I have felt so shite!

Thursday, 10 November:

Well, I didn't sleep last night, thanks to the weird sweating. I have no energy, am sore everywhere and bloody miserable.

Somehow I got myself to Motivation where I was weighed. I am down 2lbs. As soon as I got home I took to the couch and there I stayed. I have no appetite or interest in anything. It just feels like I am in some sort of health limbo. The diet is going to be well fucked up because of the antibiotics and I am on my second bottle of cough medicine.

Friday, 11 November:

Still feel crap!

Saturday, 12 November:

Still sick!

Sunday, 13 November:

My chest infection is getting worse. I can't quite believe that I can go from feeling so strong and fit, in the lead up to the marathon, to lying on a couch and being quite so ill. Certainly, I expected my body to be wrecked after it but I never thought it would be as bad as this. I am anxious to get back into my training, this is absolutely bloody frustrating.

Monday, 14 November: (Week 45)

I had to go back to the doctor. He put me on stronger antibiotics and he also had to put me on a machine, dispensing oxygen and medicine, for about ten minutes, to help me breathe more easily. I left with a week's worth of inhaler. Things better start improving now!

Tuesday, 15 November:

I went into college this morning, for about an hour, and left again, wondering why I had bothered since I still felt awful and had given in a note which excused me until Thursday. The good news is that I'm starting to cough up phleghm – it's all relative!

After spending some time thinking about it, I emailed the organisers of the Dublin Marathon to protest against the early removal of the road signs and water stations, and received, by way of reply, a cool reminder about race rules. So, nothing, I assume, is going to change there. Ah well, at least I tried.

Thursday, 17 November:

I went back to college today. Thank God! I couldn't stand being cooped up in the house any longer.

Motivation weighed me in at twenty-nine stone, so I'm down seven pounds, which is grand, I suppose, considering that I expected the antibiotics and cough bottle to mess me around a lot more than this.

Friday, 18 November:

I'm still not back at training, but I did keep myself busy this afternoon, planning out my goals for next year. It is better for my mental health if I keep thinking about moving forward.

If I serious about doing the Marathon des Sables I really have to put in a huge effort for the next sixteen months. Thinking about it brings me out in goose bumps of excitement.

Monday, 21 November (Week 46)

At last I was able to train tonight. My breathing still isn't one hundred per cent and I did feel slightly winded the whole time; however it was just wonderful to be back in the gym.

I emailed Siobhan Hogan, so I'm due back for my next interview with Ray on 6 December, giving me two weeks to recover from the antibiotics.

After the last miserable couple of weeks I have recovered my mojo. Life is good, I am back training, college is tough but going well and I am absolutely in love with my wife.

My new goal: by 17 January 2012 I will have lost another fifteen stone.

Wednesday, 23 November:

Three hours of economics and two hours of maths. Need I say more?

I'm thinking about climbing Croagh Patrick over Christmas. It will give me something to focus on over the holiday period, which could prove challenging to my diet. When you go on a diet you never stop to consider that heart-warming day, that we call Christmas.

My favourite dinner, ever, has to be my mother's Christmas dinner: turkey, ham, stuffing, roast potatoes and vegetables. However, it's not just the taste of it, I'm sure most people agree that the Christmas dinner is the only meal that has a lifetime of happy memories associated with it. I always enjoy Christmas Day, just relaxing with the family, feeling safe and comfortable. But the thought of the day without the dinner is a bit more than I can bear, at this point. I have never, not looked forward to Christmas Day and I wasn't planning on starting to now.

The amount of people who have told me that they also got sick after doing their first marathon is unreal. Why didn't anybody warn us about this? Although I know it makes sense, since you are basically asking your body to do something seriously stressfully so, of course, there has to be the possibility of dire consequences. The body is only human after all.

For me, Christmas was a bit of a worry and I felt setting myself the goal of Croagh Patrick would get me through a period that for most people would be great but for me was a little unnerving. All that being said I had a tough few weeks after the marathon, but I was coming through that and getting a chance to think about what I had done. I had spent a large part of my life giving up and the marathon was without doubt the hardest thing I had ever done, it was way harder than I ever expected and it tested me in ways I never imagined, but by keeping going I had come out the other side with a new sense of belief in myself. I felt I was a stronger person and I also had a new perspective on people and life. This may sound very profound, but when you go through something that is so hard you do take something out of it. I never expected I would take so much away from it.

Sunday, 27 November:

I went swimming this morning and totally winded myself even before doing one complete lap. Talk about frustration! I'll have to go back to the doctor's tomorrow.

Monday, 28 November: (Week 47)

The doctor put me on even stronger antibiotics, warning me that they will definitely affect the diet and may cause bloating. Terrific!

I had a math's exam today, it went okay, I suppose. Please God, I'll get 50 per cent, at least – which is the best I can hope for. I know I haven't been really working like I should because of being ill.

Today, in general, was not a good day. I'm struggling with the diet and am still below par at training. My energy levels are down so I feel exhausted and, to be honest, bloody miserable. It's like I can't stop feeling sorry for myself. All I can think about is how tired I am and how difficult everything is. This isn't me but I can't seem to snap out of it.

Wednesday, 30 November:

I got my act together and went swimming this morning after

renewing my membership. It is time to get back in the saddle regarding training and exercise. My body may not like it but if I keep pushing through I should be alright.

The fertility clinic contacted Shelly to say it could be July or August, of next year, before they call us for IUI. I think she was a bit disappointed by this but what can we do.

Thursday, 1 December:

Well, yesterday I found my positivity, but this morning I managed to blow it away again. I'm like a cut cat, thanks to weighing myself and discovering that I am up by ten pounds in just four days. I don't mind admitting that I was very near tears.

I know it wasn't going to be good news, especially after the doctor warned me, but still I didn't expect that much of a jump. Am I just going to keep getting bigger and bigger, thanks to tablets? I feel so helpless about it.

My result was confirmed when I got weighed in Motivation. I can't write anymore tonight, I'm too pissed off.

This was something that was really getting me down at this time. The problem with the ketosis diet is that it's such a fine line; your body is either in or out of ketosis, there is no middle ground. Yes, it is a great diet for losing weight fast, but when anything is introduced to your body that will take you out of ketosis – such as antibiotics – it becomes a nightmare. It makes your body pull in the water you have lost. While it is temporary, it is also soul destroying. In the game of numbers that is a diet, it really does cause a lot of self-doubt. For most people, these times are where a diet is won or lost. The week you have worked your ass off and still you put up weight, you stand and look down in bewilderment thinking, 'What has gone wrong?', but I had been here before and even though it really was testing my resolve I wasn't giving up. Even though it was very hard and I was miserable I just kept going.

Friday, 2 December:

This morning saw me back in the pool and I think my chest felt a fraction better.

I was a bit sceptical about going to training tonight, thinking I wouldn't be able for it, but, while it was tough going, it went much better than expected. Afterwards I had a good chat with Chris, which helped me, as I needed to get some stuff off my chest about where I was going and what I wanted to do, fitness wise.

Sunday, 4 December:

I feel a little better today though I am dreading Tuesday's interview with Ray. It is just so disappointing, the weight going up thanks to three courses of antibiotics, which is fair enough, I suppose. It's just that I hate sounding like I am making excuses. I feel like I am letting everyone down. Honestly, I have never felt so low, and guilty, before an interview.

Monday, 5 December: (Week 48)

This morning I had a bit of a shock when I realised that I have one week left to exams. I'll have to knuckle down, particularly with economics as I am lost at the moment. On the plus side I got back the results of my maths & stats exam: 81%, and I am very happy with that.

Tuesday, 6 December:

I got up at 5.30am to drive to Today FM. Jenny met me in reception and we had a good chat about the last couple of weeks. She gave me the good news that the show would be sticking with me until the end of my journey. I had worried that they might finish with my story in January, marking the twelve month anniversary since I contacted them. Thank goodness for that. I have come to rely on their support so much.

The interview went well, I had been nervous owing to my bad month, but Ray asked about the antibiotics and how exactly they affected the diet and my weight. The only thing I feel bad about is that I could not tell him I had been put on steroids for my chest because I was sure it would sound bad, or possibly even damaging. Maybe I'm just being paranoid.

He asked me about the Marathon des Sables and what my plans were for Christmas, and I don't feel that I explained myself very well. I was mortified with the weigh-in and it played heavily on my mind that I wasn't sitting there with a better result.

I drove back to college afterwards.

It might surprise people that when I started this process with Today FM it was pretty informal – they offered help and I accepted, which was to be the best decision I ever made. However, in times like these I always feared that they would say that it had run its course, so the reassurance offered by Jenny was fantastic and coming into Christmas was a massive comfort to keep me motivate. I had briefly hinted about the Marathon des Sables to them and I was surprised that Ray asked me about it. I knew he thought I was mad and most people still do, but for me it was about testing myself.

Wednesday, 7 December:

This week is all about study. I spent the day in library, with my head immersed in my economics and accounting books. By 4pm I was glad to escape to the gym and blow the cobwebs out of my sore brain.

We had another night out for Limerick Charity Boxing, an event I helped to set up. I sipped water for a few hours before quietly slipping away but it was a good night. God knows I needed the cheering up. So far we have raised €38,000, which is pretty impressive for something that has only been going for six months or so.

Thursday, 8 December:

I spent over an hour in UL pool, this morning, and while I could congratulate myself on my dedication I would have to be honest and admit that just maybe it was more about putting off going into college to study.

Shelly decided she would go to her college (UL) to study so I went home instead of to the library and got quite a bit of work done. I think it helps that the both of us are having exams. We understand what the other is going through.

Friday, 9 December:

I studied at home again, after my morning swim. For most of the day I felt drained, mentally, but then I went training at TriFit and felt a lot better for it. When I have a mental slump I honestly find that exercise wakes me up again, making me more alert and focused on my college work.

The TriFit Christmas party was on tonight and Chris practically ordered me to be there. I planned to go for an hour, but ended up staying for much longer than that. It was a great night and I didn't mind not drinking at all. The only hiccup was when they brought out the food I was so very, very tempted. Plates of chicken wings and cocktail sausages whizzed passed me and smelled absolutely delicious. By that stage, I could have eaten my arm. That's the thing about being on a diet, you never get used to it, particularly when you are in close proximity to the likes of tiny sausages, bite-size and perfectly cooked. I've learned that it's OK to want something, but I know it's not worth it. I was also helped by the great company so what could have felt like a big thing was a fleeting moment in a really great night.

There was an award ceremony, hosted by Chris, who presented me with a Superman tee-shirt, for the 'super effort' I have made to date. I headed home around midnight because the alcohol had started to kick in, bringing an end to sensible conversation.

Saturday, 10 December:

Today was all about economics. Shelly went to college to study while I stayed here, working right up to 9pm. I feel like I'm starting to understand economics now, which is bloody brilliant, since all term I have been really struggling with it.

At times it is hard for both Shelly and me being back at college especially as these were our first exams together. It was certainly challenging to keep everything going at the same time, but you do what you must!

The one good thing about exams is that it takes my mind off food and the diet.

Nicole is coming for a sleep-over tonight, giving Shelly and me a much needed break from worrying about our respective subjects.

Monday, 12 December: (Week 49)

Jesus Christ! What a fright I had this morning. I went swimming first thing and then headed into the college library to study for my economics exam in the afternoon. Something made me go and check the time-table, to see what time the exam was at, and there I discovered that today was the day of the accounting exam, not economics, the subject I had been studying non-stop for the past few days. I thought my heart was going to leap up my throat and onto the floor in front of me. I raced back to the library and crammed, like mad, on accounting, before heading straight in for the exam. It is hard to tell, but I think I might have got through it, although I definitely struggled to get everything done with the two hours.

I skipped training tonight and stayed in the library to study economics, and this time I am sure of exactly when and where it takes place!

A guy contacted me on Facebook. He heard me talk about the Marathon des Sables on Ray's show and wrote to tell me that the 2013 marathon was booked solid. I had written to them in September and was told that the places would not be going on sale until next June. He gave me another website for it so I've sent a second email about applying to take part.

Tuesday, 13 December:

Oh, joy! The last day of exams! I spent the morning in the library, and then went in for the economics exam which, I think, went very well. It was such a wonderful feeling to walk out of the exam hall, knowing that I was officially on my Christmas holidays.

A girl approached and started chatting to me about the exam. I hadn't a clue who she was but she obviously recognised me as someone from her class. Next year I really need to make the effort to get to know a few more people.

Wednesday, 14 December:

I am glad to say I had a lie in this morning and didn't get to UL gym until 10am. Before I went for my swim I spent twenty minutes on the exercise bike, working up a sweat. It felt so luxurious not having to think about economics, accounting and exams. My poor brain is in dire need of a break.

However, there is no denying it, no matter how much of a struggle the last couple of weeks have been, the exams proved to be a great distraction from the diet so I think I am going to be okay over the next few weeks.

I received an email from the Marathon des Sables rep in the UK, who told me that the 2013 race was full. Also they have changed agents and, apparently, I had been dealing with the old agent back in September. I thanked him for getting back to me and explained my story to him, hoping he could squeeze me in. All I can do is wait. At the very least he will put me on the reserve list, but I think it is important to have an official place for us. How can you train for something like this with just a reserve placing?

Thursday, 15 December:

I went swimming at 10am, again, this morning and the pool was quieter than normal, allowing me to enjoy my session more. Splitting the hour into three, I spent the first fifteen swimming, twenty minutes doing aqua jogging and then finished with another thirty minutes of swimming.

I had to go to a meeting today and while waiting for the person to arrive I overheard a conversation that I was not supposed to hear as it was about me, describing me as 'you can't miss him'. While I really felt low about it, I felt a little angry too and disappointed in myself. I felt I had come so far, but obviously not as far as I had thought.

On the plus side I have decided to set up a website. I met up with Niall Fitz who is giving me a hand with it. It will be a point of contact for me as I get a lot of emails which I love as I really like being in a position to offer some hope. I just wish I could do more, but if this makes it easier to contact me it will help and it will also keep people more up to date with my story and everything that is happening.

Friday, 16 December:

I still felt quite down when I woke up this morning, but then I went swimming which gave me the mental boost that I needed, as well as working off my frustrations.

When I came home I cleaned the house and fetched out the Christmas decorations, all the while thinking about how much my life has changed over the past eleven months or so. For one thing I could not have managed the cleaning this time last year, apart from the physical disability, from being so heavy, I would not have had the interest. Not that I was suicidal – I don't think I ever got that bad – but I probably stopped caring about stuff like Christmas decorations and I had gotten to the stage where I didn't care if I lived or died, with little or no curiosity about what any new day might bring. I had only two reasons for living and that was Shelly and my family.

Fast forward to today and I am lucky to have been given a second chance, albeit with lots of hard work. I love life and when I think how far I have come I get very emotional and very grateful for everything that has happened.

Yesterday was a dose of reality. At least I think that's what it was. I am going to have deal with the fact that some people will only see the 'fat man', and can I really blame them? After all, I am still over twenty-eight stone. I'm not stupid. I guess I have to take it as it comes; if people have a less than supportive reaction to me then I just have to use it to spur me on. I knew this wasn't going to be easy. Other illness, or whatever, can be hidden away for the chosen few, something I cannot do with my body. It is out there, in public, and up for general opinion. I am spent the last few weeks feeling sorry for myself. That has to stop. It is time for me to jump back into the game and finish this journey, this story of mine with style.

The MdS (Marathon des Sables) rep replied to my email, they have made four charity places available for us which is great news. The only thing is we have to commit to raising money for a charity in Africa, which is supported by MdS, and costs extra, but, so what, if it guarantees my place. I will have to find the money for my own deposit, of £2,000stg, as soon as I can, in order to secure the places.

Normally when I hear someone say the line, 'If it is meant to be, it is meant to be', it irritates the crap out of me. However, in this case, I will make an exception.

So my next move is to email everyone who had expressed an interest in doing the race with me over the past few weeks to see if they still feel the same way.

Saturday, 17 December:

So much for my pep talk yesterday. This morning was a struggle, despite the swim. I came home and watched an episode of **The Biggest Loser**, an old reliable, when it comes to kick-starting a positive attitude. It worked its usual magic on me.

Shelly's last exam was today so now, since she's on holidays too, Christmas is now officially on. I feel torn about the day itself, half dreading it and half excited about it.

Well, the responses to my email have been funny, lots of people suddenly saying that they can't do the race. On the other hand the one person that I would have expected to bail is paying her deposit on Monday, which is a huge relief. Go, Angela! I was worried that if it was just Chris and I and something happened to him I'd be on my own. I have a strong feeling that you would really need a mate beside you to do this particular race.

I had met Angela during the Dublin Marathon and after a very brief conversation she was gone. A few days later she emailed me to say 'well done', then we just kept emailing each other and I ended up telling her about the MdS. I was surprised at the time that she signed up, but knowing her better now I am not. She has become a great friend and a person who is great to talk to about what is going on as she is removed from it and gives great advice, Having other people with me would be a safety net as while Chris had said he would do it I felt a little guilty as he would be away from his family for so long.

Sunday, 18 December:

When I woke up this morning my tip-top attitude was that I was not going to mope around the house like I did yesterday. Following that brave thought I went on to have one of my very worse days in a long time. In fact I might even describe today as being the hardest day of the entire year.

I made a mistake last night. I put a post on boards.ie asking if anyone had been to the MdS and if they had any advice. Instead of training advice, which was what I was hoping for, I received far too many personal opinions about whether I could do it or not. Some people came out and said I was a fool for trying. Jesus!

Why, oh why, did I go on that bloody message board about the MdS? I wish I could forget some of the comments, but they really hit close to the bone. I find other people's negativity hard to handle. My attitude is that I would rather try and fail, than not try at all. The sensible thing is to believe that some of the contributors were coming from the point of view that they wouldn't be able to do it, so why should I? It was more about them than me.

At least I have made the important decision to eat a Christmas dinner. In other words, instead of dreading Christmas Day and feeling sorry for myself, I will eat my dinner and enjoy my day, just like everyone else. Bouncing to and fro in my head about whether or not to allow myself to indulge is soul destroying. It is just one meal and I have to see things in perspective. I don't want to feel guilty. Whatever anyone else thinks about this, I think I deserve it.

Monday, 19 December:(Week 50)

I got up and went to the gym this morning, doing twenty minutes on the bike, until my ass began to hurt, and then got into the pool, spending an hour alternating between swimming and aqua jogging. At least my body felt good after it, even if my mind didn't.

Maybe I miss the routine of college but I was just hanging, or moping, around the house when I decided to start reading Gerry Duffy's book again. It does help with motivation and God knows I have the time.

Lorraine is standing in for Chris, he went home to Australia for Christmas, and she is great, and easy on the eye, being a former Miss Limerick and Miss Ireland contestant. However, I do miss Chris getting inside my head and pushing me to the limit.

Tuesday, 20 December:

I was a man on a mission this morning, getting all my Christmas shopping done in under an hour, not that I had many people to buy for but I still think I did a really good job.

Shelly and I don't really go in for big presents so I got her favourite bottle of perfume, Jean Paul Gaultier, and I'll give her money to get herself clothes. I can never forget the name of the perfume. When we first started going out I noticed it, the fragrance is very distinctive. This was back in 2001 when we first started dating. I had to go to my cousin's wedding in Valencia, Spain, with the family, and we were flying back from Barcelona Airport when I snuck off to duty free to buy Shelly a present. I hadn't much experience of buying presents for girlfriends, but it struck me I was in a good place to buy her a bottle of her favourite perfume. It was only when I was faced with rows and rows of perfumes that I realised I hadn't a clue what it was called. So I stood there, waiting for inspiration, feeling lost and bewildered. After a couple of panicked minutes I decided to pick any one of them up when I suddenly caught a whiff of Shelly. I turned to see what looked like a pair of models, a young guy and his girlfriend, walk by me. Without thinking – because if I had stopped to think there is no way I would have been able to talk to this gorgeous pair like this – I asked the girl, who was simply stunning, 'Excuse me, but my girlfriend wears the same perfume as you and I don't know the name. Could you help me, please?' Maybe it was the Irish accent or the genuine look of worry on my face, whatever it was she smiled kindly and took me by the arm, leading me straight to the bottles on display, telling me that my girlfriend, 'was a lucky lady!' Her partner gave me an equally stunning smile and winked, as if to say, 'Good man, yourself!'

After shopping I did a good session in UL.

Cllr Joe Leddin rang me this afternoon to ask would I do the Great Limerick Run. He's on the organising committee. I told him I wasn't sure and he asked could we meet over the holiday to chat about it. I just don't want to go through what I did in Dublin with no signs or water ... I must be mad entertaining doing a second marathon, but now I know I can so why not?

Now I feel I am getting in the Christmas spirit. At last!

Wednesday, 21 December:

Siobhan Hogan rang me this morning to ask if I would be available to talk to Ray tomorrow morning, on the phone. That was a nice surprise.

I had my last TriFit session today because they close for Christmas until the second week in January, which is a pain but I have learned a lot in the past few months from Chris so I will just keep going with training.

Thursday, 22 December:

Ray rang about 11am, wanting to wish me a Happy Christmas and offer some support. I think he realises that the Christmas season is going to be a bit rough for me.

I paid my deposit for the MdS, so it is official. I am going to be part of the 2013 race. The enormity of this hit me once the bank transfer went through. This is going to be interesting, at the very least.

There is something wrong with the car so Dad and I brought it around to Pat Gorey, who let us use his ramp. This is worrying; I think it might be something to do with the gear box which could be expensive.

Friday, 23 December:

Okay, so now I am really excited about Christmas and am very much looking forward to eating my dinner.

Saturday, 24 December:

Talk about mood swings. Today, Christmas Eve, got quite emotional for me and Shelly. Christmas is all about children and I fell into the pit today, wondering if we would ever have any or what to do if we couldn't. I know it eats Shelly up inside.

I spent the evening with Nicole, who is hyper about tomorrow. It was a bittersweet evening for me, I love being with her, but tonight I found myself wishing I had my own child to buy presents for.

At any rate I am really looking forward to tomorrow.

Sunday, 25 December:

Well, after all my worrying, I had a lovely day. We got up and had breakfast; I had my normal protein drink, but then had a small bowl of Cheerios. We went down to Mam's where there were loads going on, with visitors and presents being unwrapped.

Dinner was spectacular though I didn't eat much. I had a little helping of everything and stopped eating when I felt full. After that we sat around chatting for hours, relaxing in front of the television. Shelly and I returned home at 9pm where I thoroughly enjoyed a cup of tea and a turkey sandwich. I'd go as far as to say that it was truly divine!

So I am delighted I made the decision to eat. I didn't touch any rubbish and remained disciplined regarding quantity. It is great to know I can trust myself around food – especially on Christmas Day.

Monday, 26 December:(Week 51)

I was back to normality today, regarding the diet. It is such a pity that UL isn't open as I would have loved to swim after all the turkey yesterday.

The weather reports for Wednesday are looking gloomy, but I'm still hoping I can climb Croagh Patrick.

Tuesday, 27 December:

Shelly has gone home, to Tipperary, for a few days, I dropped her to the train station. I hated seeing her go. On the plus side, however, UL reopened today so I went for a swim in the afternoon. It really helps with the diet, to be able to do exercise. Unfortunately the pool was quite busy with people cutting into my lane with wilful abandonment. One guy in particular had me wanting to scream.

When I came out of the shower and was heading to the cubicles, in just my swimming trunks, a very pretty girl, clad in a bikini, stopped to chat to me. I was mortified and then rude, I shut the door to the cubicle in her face as I couldn't forget I was practically naked.

I came home and sank in front of the television, watching one bad film after another. When I felt my mood beginning to really plunge I got up and packed for tomorrow's climb, though the weather reports have not improved. Nevertheless I am going to drive up to it, no matter what, for my own piece of mind. Rob (my brother) is coming with me. I couldn't sit in the house, looking out the window, wondering if I should go or not. It is best I drive up and then make my decision, knowing that I was willing to do it, right to the end.

Mam rang after 8pm to tell me that Rob won €50,000 on a scratch card! Unable to believe it I went down to the house. It was the most complicated scratch card I have ever seen, but yes, he really had won the money. Miracles do happen!

Wednesday, 28 December:

I got up at 5am and Rob and I drove to Westport. The weather wasn't too bad and I started to think that we might get to do the climb but then, just outside Westport, the wind really picked up.

The road to Croagh Patrick is along the coast, which would be marvellous had it been a summer's day. Instead Rob and I saw the sea smashing off the rocks, sending water splashing across the road in front of us, which I think we both knew was a bad sign. I stopped at the foot of the mountain and as we were sitting there the car was rocking back and forth. Again, not a good sign.

To our credit we got out of the car and tried to push forward, against the wind. It was very disappointing but it would have been risking life and limb to have attempted a climb in that weather. I knew it was a long shot but in saying that, I was glad that I had driven up to the base. After all I can't control the weather and that was the only thing that prevented me from doing it. So, it wasn't a wasted drive. To be honest I felt it was a bit of a victory in itself to have gone all the way to Westport. I would have felt worse if I had stayed home and imagined that the weather might have been too bad.

I dropped Rob home and went for a swim at UL.

I knew full well two days earlier that we wouldn't be able to climb, it but I knew I had to make the effort and go. I wasn't giving up and while it may sound crazy to some people, to me crazy would having been sitting on a couch saying, 'Ah well, no.' The new me would at least give it a go. On the plus side I got to spend some time with Rob and we had a laugh.

Thursday, 29 December:

I had a great session in UL this morning. I even went up to the running track and walked hard for thirty minutes.

Shelly came home this afternoon. Thank goodness!

This evening I sat down and began to sort out what I am going to do in 2012. A couple of ideas have been running through my mind, over the last while, so I want to write them down here and commit to them in print.

Okay, so I am going to do a 5k run in April. I hope it will be with Ray, and the radio show, but if not I will find a substitute.

In June I am thinking about doing the Tri Athy, Ireland's fastest triathlon course, though I am unwilling to be definite about this until nearer the time, because of the strict time limits regarding completing it. I want to know I can do it before I sign up for it. There is another big race that is catching my eye, the Gaelforce adventure race in August, which runs for the entire day and involves cycling, running, hiking and kayaking. It sounds like great fun. Then, in October, I want to knock between three and four hours off my time for the Dublin marathon.

After that it will be all about training for the Marathon des Sables. A tough and challenging sixteen months ahead, but I am really looking forward to it.

Sunday, 30 December:

Jesus! Who would have guessed that my drive to Mayo would have such a positive effect on me? I feel great and absolutely back on track with the diet and training. UL opened at 11am and I was practically the first one through the door.

My aim for the rest of this year, that is, the next two days, is to finish the year as I lived it. Therefore, I will be eating only broccoli, cauliflower and chicken, training very hard and enjoying my ever-changing life, before starting 2012 in the same manner.

Saturday, 31 December:

I finished the year with a good swim and stiff walk around the UL campus.

New Year's Eve, and while I don't really want this year to end I can't but be excited about what I will do in 2012. I know I still have a long road ahead of me but I have to appreciate how much I have changed since this time last year.

Nicole is staying with us tonight and I will be welcoming in the New Year with a protein drink, although I am having steak for dinner and am really looking forward to it.

Happy New Year!

Sunday, 1 January 2012

The New Year is like a blank canvas and it is up to me the picture I will paint. I take the time here to bid farewell to 2011, with all the wonderful memories and the equally wonderfully people I was lucky to meet and get to know.

This time next year I will not be overweight. And anything else that happens along the way will be a bonus.

Monday, 2 January: (Week 52)

I hate the way that everything stops for Christmas. Tomorrow the pool and gym will be back to normal and I cannot wait.

I went swimming this afternoon which wasn't a great idea

since the pool was crammed with a swimming club for kids. There were loads of parents sitting around the pool which I personally found off-putting. I'm sure they should have been sitting up in the gallery. I also saw a lot of people ignore the signs and take photographs with their mobile phones, which is just not allowed anymore. The whole experience pissed me off!

Still, it was a perfect day, regarding the diet and my motivation. I'm definitely back on track.

Tuesday, 3 January:

Swallowing my scepticism, I met with Joe Leddin and the director of the Great Limerick Run, John Cleary tonight. To my delight it was a very enjoyable and productive meeting. Initially, they were just interested in invited me along to take part in the run, which was grand except for the fact that I was still a bit raw about what happened at the Dublin Marathon. Fortunately I felt able to raise my concerns about signage and water stations which stimulated a great discussion on how to improve things for the Limerick race. Their open attitude made me feel newly positive about walking big races as they really listened to me and nodded along with my ideas, as well as presenting some great ones of their own.

Basically, I am going to do this marathon and it is going to be opened up to include a 5.5hr plus category that will have a cut off time of ten hours. This means that people can walk the race if they want to. So, for ten hours, there will be water stations. Actually they said there would be water available until every single competitor had finished the race. The 5.5hr category will commence at 8am, an hour before the runners take off, meaning that there is a better chance of being surrounded by other competitors for longer.

The finish line will remain until 5pm, as will the medical treatments behind the finish line. They are going to follow my own training up until the marathon and Chris will put all the details of my training up on their website, should anyone else like to copy what I'm doing. In this way I feel that the walkers, like myself, will feel very much included in the day. No one is going to be walking for hours by themselves, wondering if they are on the right road or when they are going to be lucky enough to be offered a drink of water.

I am really excited. It's just a small thing, I suppose, but I really want to be able to help others, to use my experience to make things a little easier for someone else. And this, I feel, is a perfect example: competing in the Dublin Marathon, experiencing the setbacks, if that's not too strong a word, and then using that knowledge to improve something like the Great Limerick Race. I am so grateful to Joe and John for giving me this opportunity.

Thursday, 5 January:

Okay, I am not the most confident of people but on a day like this even I have to admit that I can rock! Motivation had to ring me to come in to be weighed because I had completely forgotten it was Thursday. I am down thirteen stone four pounds. I just might make fourteen stone within the next twelve days. Yeah!

They also told me it was time to move onto a different nutrition plan because they feel that I have been on this medical diet for long enough. This took me by surprise, but after they explained it to me I am happy enough. No, let's say that I am delighted, and why wouldn't I be, since I am now allowed to include foods like cereals, bread, potatoes, rice, porridge, fruit and a selection of vegetables in my day. The quantities are tiny, but no matter, it is going to make the diet so much easier to stick to.

I am going to Tesco tomorrow with a shopping list that will be as varied as I like.

Friday, 6 January:

I had a second meeting with the Great Limerick Run people which left me on a high. So, briefly, there is going to be a five-hour plus category, aimed at walkers and runners alike. It will begin an hour before the real runners, who will have to pass us by. I don't think this happens in any other marathon. The walkers do the first half of the race and then, as we approach the city again, we will automatically be taking part in a half-marathon, with the crowd stationed around that particular starting line, egging us on. We will also be linked up with the 5k run, which starts later in the day.

The lads want the water stations open until 6pm and the signs will remain up all day. They are meeting with the Gardaí, to see about keeping the finish line open until 6pm. If that isn't possible they are going to set up a special mini-marathon finish line, which means that everyone will get to cross it.

I am going to start writing a weekly blog, for their website, to help people prepare for the five hour-hour plus category. I really hope that people join in with me and suggested to the lads that Chris and I could set up a walk/run session every Sunday, until the race, for anybody who might like to train with me. I'll be out doing it anyway, so I could do with the company.

It is such a buzz that they want someone like me, not only taking part in their race, but also asking me for my suggestions to make it a good event for everybody. When I think of how I practically walked in the shadows while doing the 5k in Cork, hoping no one would know I was taking part in the race. This would have unimaginable to me back then.

Jesus! I was so pissed off tonight. Molly ate one of my €140 runners. I had to throw the pair in the bin. Venting my frustration I went on Facebook and wrote about it. Lots of sympathetic reactions calmed me down but then Dorothy, from the Tri and Run sports shop, in Mullingar, offered me a new pair to say 'well done' for all my hard work.

I feel very blessed with the people my 'journey' has brought me in contact with. When I think of how cynical I had grown about the public in general, when I was at my heaviest, the very same public who have supported me and then come through for me when I needed it. Thank you, Dorothy!

Saturday, 7 January:

I found this quote this morning from the Russian write Leo Tolstoy, who wrote **War and Peace**, 'Everyone thinks of changing the world, but no one thinks of changing himself'. I'd like to think that this doesn't apply to me. Not only do I want to change myself, I absolutely believe that I **am** changing myself.

Tomorrow's weather forecast is good – thank God! – since Shelly and I are going to climb Croagh Patrick. This time last year, I don't think either of us would have believed we would ever be doing something like this together.

I got myself a copy of **Run Fat Bitch Run** by Ruth Field. It sounds interesting, but whether it has anything for me is another thing.

Sunday, 8 January:

Shelly and I were on the road for Westport by 7am. We were looking forward to the first sighting of Croagh Patrick, after Castlebar, howovor it was covered over by grey cloud. My heart sank a bit but I kept driving.

About twenty minutes later we arrived in the car-park and found quite a few people preparing to climb. The weather wasn't too bad; it was neither freezing nor raining though the clouds were still hanging low. Unfortunately, the Visitors' Centre was closed which meant we couldn't avail of the walking poles that I had been told were vital to doing the climb. We headed to the base, passing the steps leading up to a statue of Saint Patrick, to begin the ascent up the rocky path. At this point I was suddenly impressed with how big the mountain was.

I had Shelly walk in front of me so I could keep an eye on her. It was bloody hard. I mean, I wasn't expecting it to be easy but neither did I realise how broken the path would be. Stretching my legs up over stones and rocks, I needed to take giant steps, making me feel like I was taking part in a particularly tough squat, or lunging session, and it was knocking the shit out of me. I didn't imagine I would have to constantly watch where I placed my feet to make sure I didn't stumble. Several other climbers overtook us, while we kept to our relatively-comfortable pace.

We climbed for a good while before stopping to take our first break, when we saw that the mountain was completely covered by a thick cloud, making it impossible to see the climbers who had passed us most recently. Taking off again the climb got steeper and steeper, sucking the life out of my lungs and legs. After a while I had to stop every now and then, to rest, because I was experiencing dizziness, giving me time to fret over going into the thick cloud and also to notice how high up I was.

I dislike heights, but somehow I hadn't appreciated that this might present a problem for today. However, I have no problem admitting that I began to feel plain scared as we climbed higher and higher, but I kept pushing myself forward after Shelly. I'm guessing that we climbed three quarters up the mountain's ridge when I began to take stock of the situation. We had reached what appeared to be the beginning of an even steeper climb and the clouds had swept in around us like a thick, dark blanket, preventing us from seeing either the top of the mountain or the car-park below.

Don't get me wrong, it was both beautiful and peaceful, and we decided to keep going. I told myself that the good thing about going up was that I didn't have to look down. I felt the ground sucking the energy out of me, but maybe this was my terror that I was trying to hold at bay. At this point I was climbing and doing my best to ignore a steep drop to our right. We kept going, me pushing myself through my fear, through a mist of cloud. It was like a dream, with no visible end in sight. Eventually we reached the place where the path flattened out before the final climb to the summit. It was time, I felt, to make a decision one way or the other.

I couldn't see more than forty feet or so, in front of me, and told Shelly that I thought it might be too dangerous to continue. There were people ahead of us but that didn't give me any comfort. It's not everyday you find yourself high up on a mountain with your loved one, surrounded by dark cloud, and having to think whether or not to give into ego and go for the top, just to say you did it, or make a responsible decision solely based on the fact that you are unsure what **might** happen should you keep heading upwards. I went with my gut feeling that we should turn around for home, but it wasn't easy, since I **did** want to be able to say I had reached the top. Nevertheless, at the same time, I was not willing to risk injury to Shelly or myself, which Shelly would have had to deal with.

It's now 7pm and as I sit here writing this, I know I made the right decision, despite the fact I was really disappointed with not completing the task I set myself. As it was, the descent was a lot scarier than I had expected. Jesus! If I was afraid going up, I was utterly shitting myself on the way back down, because it was then it became clear that all either of us had to do was miss our footing and go skidding off to God knows where. We kept to a slow, careful pace that was agonising to maintain. I don't think I've ever been so thankful to see a statue of a saint. There was St Patrick, at the foot of the mountain, awaiting our return, welcoming us back to level ground; I fought the urge to hug him.

Monday, 9 January: (Week 53)

Things went back to normal today, mostly. I swam and went to college, first day of the new term. Then I came home and weighed myself. Last Thursday I was minus thirteen stone and four pounds, today I am minus twelve stone and thirteen pounds, so I am up by five pounds. This, I know, is because I am now eating 'real' food, though in small portions and, of course, it was going to make a difference. The diet has been made so much easier, with the introduction of variety, and I am very careful with the amounts. However, it is never easy when the scales go up instead of down.

Tuesday, 10 January:

Caroline Crawford, from the **Evening Herald**, rang me today for an interview. I have adopted a new attitude towards journalists. I understand the situation better now, if they want a story they will write about me whether I speak to them or not, so I am going to start responding to them, or, at least, the professional ones, the ones who want to cover a real story about me. I enjoyed talking to Caroline, we covered a lot of ground.

Being back at college definitely makes the day go quicker and is a good distraction from thinking about the diet.

I'm getting stuck into **Run Fat Bit Run**. It's making me think a lot. Obviously there are parts that hold no significance for me, but she did get me thinking about swimming. Lately, when I swim I forget I am actually swimming, or performing an exercise to keep fit. Instead, I feel that I am simply 'being', when I swim. My head clears and I just enjoy the moment, and usually feel a lot better afterwards. I hope, at some stage, to feel that way about running.

Wednesday, 11 January:

God! I was flying in the pool this morning and didn't want to get out of it but I had to since I had a 9am class. Next I got the results of my Economics exam: 74 per cent. What an unexpected result!

This had been a very good day, indeed.

Then I found this quote which stopped me in my tracks before getting me all fired up. It says so much in just a few words: **I may not be there yet, but I'm closer than I was yesterday.**

Thursday, 12 January:

Returning to early morning starts has been a pleasant return to normality. I only had two hours of classes today and came home early to study.

I had planned to go for a good walk but my heel is giving me trouble. TriFit's Emlyn is going to have a look at it for me on Monday and, in the meantime, he gave me some exercises to do, including standing barefoot on a cold golf ball, which felt heavenly and really got at the muscle.

Friday, 13 January:

It's an unlucky day for some, Friday the 13th, but not for me! The diet is going so well at the moment that I hardly give it a minute's thought.

Two incidents today that made me laugh. First, a friend of mine, Gary Wilmott, rang me to say that the girl who approached me all those weeks ago, at the UL pool, works with him. She read a comment that I left on Gary's Facebook page and asked him how he knew me. He told her we were friends and she explained how she saw me at the pool and felt star struck (God only knows why!), and came over to talk to me. Maybe she didn't notice that I practically closed the cubicle door in her face, out my sheer embarrassment.

The editor from the **Evening Herald** rang me about Caroline's interview as he needed to check something because he believed it was a mistake, 'Gary, I think Caroline got muddled up in her details. She wrote here that you were forty-one stone but I presume she meant thirty-one stone?'

He sounded utterly shocked when I told him that Caroline was right, and that I had lost twelve and a half stone in the past year.

Saturday, 14 January:

Well, it is one year to the day that Ray D'Arcy read out my email on the Fix-it Friday feature. I'm about to head out to UL to train and I will deal with this anniversary on my return.

There was an **Operation Transformation** walk on at UL, which meant there were loads of people around and I did feel slightly uncomfortable when I felt I was being watched, as I went through my stuff on the running track, nevertheless it was a good session.

Okay, so. This time last year I sent, in Shelly's name, the all-important email into the Ray D'Arcy Show, out of desperation. I was depressed, lacking in self-confidence and had turned into a recluse due to the fact that when I left the house people looked at me like I was a piece of shit. I was bitter, full of hatred and anger for the world I lived in. My health reflected how bad I felt on the inside, with constant fatigue, numerous skin problems, no colour in my face, sore back, sore joints...well, pretty much sore everything. My wife, by necessity, if not choice, was my carer since I was severely limited in what I could do. She did everything for me, for the house, and for herself.

Here I am, twelve months later. I have lost almost thirteen stone and while this has obviously resulted in massive physical changes that is only one of the positive aspects that have occurred. Yes, I am a lot healthier today, but also I am happier, much more confident, more out-going and hate staying in the house when I could be out walking or swimming.

My relationships with people have vastly improved. Because I have lost that anger and bitterness, I am less judgemental and easier, I imagine, to get along with. My relationship with Shelly is back to where it should be. We enjoy all the simple things that other couples would have taken for granted, such as her being able to get her arms all the way around me when she hugs me. When I used to wallow in negativity, I do my best to avoid it now, knowing that I can chase away the cobwebs with an hour's swim.

I have met and made some great friends, most notably Chris, my personal trainer, who has been such an enormous help that I don't think I could do justice to him here.

Now there are still improvements to be made. In college I am still a bit of a loner. I avoid eye contact with people because I am so used, from before, to staring at the ground as I walked along the streets, not wanting to see anyone look at me. While my confidence has definitely grown, it can wobble from time to time, throwing me off.

My fitness and general health will, I hope, continue to get better. There are those unsightly areas, on my body, where the skin sags and I pray that they can be fixed somewhere down the line.

I have a big year ahead of me, with some big goals to reach for. Whether or not I complete everything I want to, at least, try my best.

What a year! To my mind, I can break it down into four important waves, after the initial start, which is still very surreal. Firstly, when I took up with the charity boxing guys, I discovered that I really enjoyed training with others in a structured environment with professional coaches. Secondly, at my sister Orla's wedding, in July, I met up with relatives who hadn't seen me in a while and received much-needed confirmation that I was definitely losing weight and on the road to change. I felt good in myself and was growing in confidence, which was the real measure of where I was in this process. Thirdly, meeting and working with Chris, who worked on both my fitness and instilling me with self-confidence, and lastly the Dublin City Marathon, where I received new kind of 'looks', of respect and camaraderie; it was harder than I ever imagined yet it gave me a new sense of belief in myself and became a very interesting life lesson for me.

At the beginning of this year my wife could not hug me properly, seats belts were impossible, as well as running with my niece, Nicole, in the park and I could not wipe my own bum without the use of a special wand – which was the singularly most embarrassing fact about being over forty stone. By the end of the year I had lost thirteen stone, was a new man who loved life, but still had a long way to go.

CHRIS DELOOZE TALKS ABOUT GARY'S TRAINING REGIME

What were your first impressions of Gary and the journey that you felt was ahead of him?

He was bigger than I expected him to be, having been asked by a mutual friend for exercises that a big man could do in safety. When I saw him for the first time I realised I would have to reassess the exercises.

I was in awe of the challenge ahead of him, and had absolute admiration for his determination. In a way he was my challenge, pushing me to extend my own capabilities as a personal trainer, in order to help him more.

You had absolutely no problem in supporting his marathon bid, can you tell me why you were so sure immediately?

As a personal trainer I would never want to stop someone from doing what they believe they can do. However, I was a little worried about Gary doing the marathon and suggested that he try shorter distances first but his mind was made up. Once I realised that, I went from 'Should he do it?' to 'This is how we're going to do it!', and went into injury-prevention mode

Do you think that anyone else could do what Gary has done/is doing, or does Gary just have the necessary qualities to work at completely transforming his life? If there are necessary qualities, can you tell me what they are?

He certainly is special. His frame of mind was what got him on this journey and has kept him there. When someone wants to transform their life they need a bigger reason than just losing weight. Gary wanted to become a father so this was the route he took. Things like marathons were just a step in the right direction toward living a healthier and happier life. After all, a marathon is just a day on your feet. It's all about attitude.

What's the biggest thing that somebody like Gary has to face, to start training themselves and their eating to lose lots of weight?

You have to first change your mind-set, your psychological attitude to life and yourself. Gary's first challenge was a mental one, and he overcame it with flying colours. He set out goals for himself, which are a great way to stay motivated. Again it's all about your reasons for wanting to change; they have to be bigger than the excuse to stay exactly how you are. Losing weight is a short-term goal; you must want to change your life long-term for the better.

Because being positive and self-confident is so important I have to recommend getting a personal trainer or someone who will keep you motivated during the bad days. Anyone embarking on a journey like this will need constant support, and from someone who knows what they're doing, who can instil 'mental power', that is, can help give you the belief in yourself, to keep going forward every single day.

Can you describe your particular approach to Gary and what made you chose those exercises/sessions?

Following a full assessment I worked with Gary one-on-one for six months before deciding that he was ready to join a class. Again, I had to realise that he recognised he was ready for the class too, so it was as much about his good mental attitude as anything else.

Regarding exercise it was all about keep his heart rate consistent (between 155 – 160 bpm) and keeping him on his feet, in preparation for walking all day for a marathon.

We had to work first on his joints, making his hips, knees and shoulders flexible.

Do you have any particular philosophy/wise words for someone like Gary who has broken their diet and is feeling hopeless about themself again?

Just turn up! You need support, so if you are having a bad day, do not cancel your exercise appointment. No matter what you've done, or eaten, you will need your trainer, or whoever you have chosen to turn to for support, to help you get past it.

I also suggest putting motivational stuff on the back of your bathroom door. Do you notice that when you're in a public toilet, you always remember, for whatever reason, the piece of graffiti that you've just read in the cubicle? So, do out something, a quote or whatever, and stick it to the back of your own door, for you to read over and over again.

For someone who is just starting out with exercise, and is

very overweight and unfit, is there a particular activity they should start with, like walking, or would swimming be better? What amount of time should they give a session and how often should they do it?

See your doctor first, before you do anything else! Your heart never lies; therefore it has to be monitored to show you exactly where you need to be.

Make a routine for your exercise, an hour that can never be taken away from you, and stick to it no matter what. Regarding exercise I firmly believe that you never do the same session twice. For instance, if you take up walking, don't do the same walk day after day. Vary your direction so that you can encounter walking uphill etc, which your usual walk mightn't incorporate. One road/path can prove more of a walk than another.

Make sure you eat a nutritional diet that takes into consider the exercise you are doing. I don't believe in cutting out carbohydrates, it's a matter of eating them at the right time of day, in conjunction with your exercise routine.

What do you think of Gary's journey to date? You must have seen him on rough days, watched him throw up after an exhausting session, maybe had to keep pumping him with confidence that he could keep going? How much, in your opinion, has he changed – body-wise and personality-wise?

The phenomenal change in his body shape is proof that everything is working. The journey to changing his body has also led to a massive change in his head. Gary has completely transformed himself. He can never go back to who he was, when he was over forty-one stone. He is on a healthy diet and exercise regime for life, and it, in turn, is getting him the life he wants, fatherhood, a growing self-confidence, and the ability to do marathons or whatever else he chooses. He can fit under a seat belt, can do sit-ups and his wife can hug him properly. All these seemingly small accomplishments were all parts of the reason he decided to lose weight and get fit.

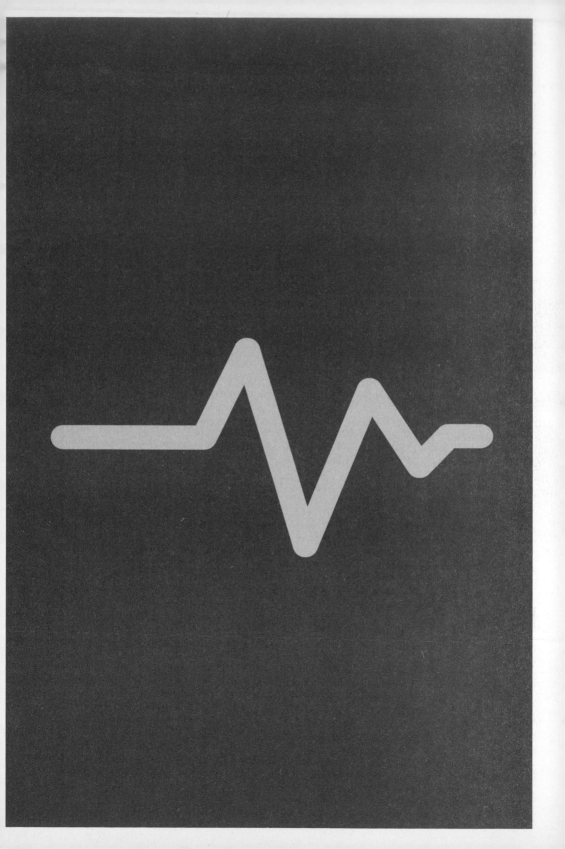

PART

THREE

CHAPTER SEVEN

2012 – YEAR TWO

This year has brought with it many more changes, a lot of highs and some lows. My website was up and running and people were starting to write to me about their weight problems and how they impacted on their life. I can't offer people much advice, unfortunately, but I believe that just having somebody in the same situation to turn to is a way for people to talk about their situation without judgment. On the 17 January I weighed in at twenty-eight stone one pound; in a year I had lost thirteen stone two pounds and while that was good, the change in me mentally was far greater.

Out of the blue I was contacted by a publisher, wanting me to write a book about my story. Now, that is something I would not have foreseen in a million years. Keeping a diary was a way to keep track of the madness; initially some of the things that happened were very unexpected and the diary was just to keep track of the day to day developments in my life. Over time it became a lot more – it became a confidant; also I could look back and see the change in my attitude.

A book, however, is completely different. I spent some time thinking about it before I agreed to sign the contract. I still can't believe anybody wants to read my story, much like the press attention, the *Ray D'Arcy Show* and even the people who have such kind comments for me, I can't see why people have any interest in my story as for me it is just my life. But if my story can help one person then it is worth telling.

I wrote in the diary, and I repeat it here, that I genuinely want to be able to help others who are struggling or were struggling with their own body weight. Plus I chose to study marketing because I have an idea that I might like to do something good in that department, regarding the marketing and labelling of food. A book, I felt, could represent a big start on both those paths.

Through the website I receive quite a lot of emails from people wanting to lose weight and make a change in their life, which I know can be a frightening prospect. To initiate a personal transformation you need to place a lot of trust in yourself and in the future. It can take a while to reach that point and admit that now is the time for action, and drag yourself mentally out of your comfort zone.

This is quite a typical email, and unfortunately so:

Dear Gary,

Firstly I am so glad you have created your website. I can only imagine the amount of people you will help by allowing them to follow your journey. I know only too well what it is like to experience being severely overweight and what it can do to the body, but more importantly what it can do to the person. I can honestly say I have not been living my life for so long now that I can hardly remember what it is like to live life to the full. I have practically been in hiding apart from going to work, and have not been out with friends or even seen some of my relatives in years because I am so self-conscious about my weight. At this stage I have completely run out of excuses to avoid get-togethers.

Thank goodness for my job or I'd probably never leave the house. It is so hard to explain this to people who could never understand what this feels like, and why should they? Truth be told I wish I didn't understand what it is like to experience these feelings of complete worthlessness especially for something that is completely within my control.

When I look at your website I feel such a strong tie to what you are doing. I would never admit it to anyone, for fear of what they might think, but one of my goals is to complete a marathon. You are such an inspiration. I know how daunting it must have been when you first started out on your journey, and can only imagine how it must feel to be finally fulfilling your potential. Equally, I know deep down inside of me I have lots of potential and am capable of being so much more than I am.

As I say this email is not unique. There are plenty of people out there who feel that they are a joke in the community. Why is it that so many overweight people feel their only option is to write to radio shows or apply to take part in television programmes? Something is wrong, don't you think?

This country was so quick to bring in the smoking ban, why are we so lax about the obesity issue? If you are an overweight person wanting, or needing, to lose weight there are a few options, and those there are fall mostly between the health service and private weight loss companies, none of which are that great. Going to a doctor or a dietician may simply lead to diet pills. I have taken these and they are not nice. When your weight becomes a serious problem you are referred to the National Obesity Clinic, in Loughlinstown, where a gastric band may be fitted to reduce the size of your stomach and, therefore, the size of your appetite. Why there is only one obesity clinic in Ireland for such a widespread problem is baffling. The waiting list is somewhere between eighteen and twenty-four months, the operation costs something like €35,000, and about two are performed each week.

What I dislike about the diet companies is that some of them lack formal nutritional qualifications, the very subject that people like me, need to know more about.

After all I've been through, I can't help thinking how much cheaper and more productive someone like Chris would be, as a pill-free, surgery-free alternative. Look at the weight-loss TV programmes, they work don't they? Personal trainers and nutritionists show off what can be achieved through old-fashioned exercise and healthy eating. Why is this sort of treatment not made more readily available to obese people? The system in Ireland is just not working for a lot of sufferers out there.

Thanks to my own personal experience combined with what I'm learning in college, I've put together my ideas on the subject. Allow me to get out my soapbox and stand on it.

The government needs to regulate the food industry. Packaging should declare all nutritional ingredients within the product and not just a percentage. You might have noticed the labels on most items: for example a 200 gramme bar of chocolate will only show information relating to 100 grammes. I've already written about a labelling system that would differentiate between genuine healthy foods and not so genuine. Regarding diet products, I think they should be subjected to tighter controls, and their promises should be scientifically proven.

The government should monitor advertising from the fast food and fizzy drinks industries. For instance I disagree with them being allowed to sponsor sporting events as it's a misleading association. On television these products should only be advertised at a certain time of the day, like alcohol.

Staying with on screen advertising, more people die from obesity-related illness than in road accidents, yet look at the amount of time that is given to those – albeit necessary – shock-tactic ads warning against drink-driving and speeding. Where are the same types of advertisements warning against being heavily overweight?

There should be way more pro-active media coverage on the subject of obesity, with healthy eating and exercise being advocated as a lifestyle choice. Tips should be aired about how to make little changes that mean a lot in terms of improving your health. The national broadcasters can get more involved here. Each January RTÉ shows the hugely-popular show *Operation Transformation*, which lasts until March, after that there is nothing for the thousands of people who have watched the show and turned up at the associated events. And what about cookery programmes that focus on healthy recipes, aimed at people wanting to lose weight?

Kids need to be encouraged to eat properly and exercise. Couldn't they learn about nutrition, as well as health and fitness in school, from an early age? Fizzy drinks and sweets should not be sold in schools. Also, regarding sports in schools I wonder if there is too much focus on team sports, which wouldn't suit everybody. There should be a wider diversity of sports available to school kids.

There needs to be an overhaul in the education of doctors and nurses regarding patients who are obese, as well as an overhaul in relation to hospital food. It is crazy that while you are sick in hospital you can have a fry-up for breakfast. Shouldn't this be the place where you learn the benefits of following a healthier diet? Doctors might think about prescribing exercise instead of pills, because it is so much more beneficial, especially, I think, in relation to treating depression.

A lot of people around the country give their time freely to coach their local football team and so on. I believe that anyone involved in sports should have to undergo basic training in sports science and nutrition and there should be tax benefits made available to them, to encourage them to further their education in these areas; these people are assets to society and should be treated accordingly.

These are all very simple ideas; yes, I know they cost money to implement, but if the situation doesn't improve we are going to have a huge amount of unhealthy people over the next ten or twenty years, who will surely cause the county more expense in the long run. It is not just excess weight that I'm talking about, it is heart disease, diabetes and a host of other weight-associated problems. As far as I see it, it really is down to the government to bring about a change through helping us access the right information, by regulating the food and drink industry through to ensuring fair and transparent advertising. Any company that doesn't comply could be taxed, forcing them to up the prices of their products.

Obesity, as a national affliction, is not going to disappear without something being done nationally. It needs to be addressed at several levels and it will benefit society. If I can do it, anybody can; they just need help and support like I had, what would I have cost the health system in years to come had I not taken responsibility?

* * *

My biggest struggle, this year, was when I put back on weight after 'real' food, including bread, was re-introduced into my diet. Mentally I struggled with this and worried if I really should be eating stuff like bread and cereal. I wanted to be healthy, to make the best decision for my body, but no way did I want to start putting on weight again. Of course it was my body pulling in water from the carbohydrates and sugar, and I had to tell myself that it was a necessary phase until my insides got used to the varied ingredients.

Meanwhile I was wondering if it was time to part from the Motivation Weight Clinic. My indecisiveness, in relation to this, weighed heavily in my mind. It wasn't easy, but then big decisions never are. They had worked wonders. I received a lovely email from a guy who saw me on Brendan O'Connor's show, last year, and, as a result, joined Motivation, losing almost five stone with them. The thing is, I was just as concerned about keeping fit and building muscle in place of fat, as with losing weight so – excuse the pun – I began to be convinced that I had outgrown Motivation's brief on me, which was solely about dropping pounds. However, they were part of my weekly routine and for weeks I put off making the break from them, because it was slightly terrifying to cut myself loose, and I didn't want to appear ungrateful to Today FM either. I finally made the break one Thursday in March.

Change can be very hard, especially when you have had success with a plan, but while I had completely changed all other aspects of my life, with Motivation I hadn't changed fully when it came to food. Today FM I found a very highly-recommended nutritionist, Nichola Forrest. As soon as I met her, I knew I had made the right decision and so we set about finding a diet that would allow me to keep exercising while losing fat and, most importantly, to find a balance in my diet that I could use forever.

Nichola told me that her husband was a triathlete and she was sporty herself, which laid any doubts I may have had to rest. Describing my current diet and training regime, I explained that I wanted to make long-term changes. Yes, I still wanted to lose weight, but I was also focused on training for marathons, and such like, and needed the energy from my food to perform as best as I could. I told her about my goal to compete in the MdS, and was comforted when she didn't baulk or make any sound of surprise at this ambition. In fact, she assured me that in order to stay focused on losing so much weight I needed big goals to work towards accomplishing such a big task.

She made small changes to my diet, which she tweaks from time to time, including cutting out grains after she discovered they didn't suit me at all. Her attitude is about making small and frequent changes, achieving results through trial and error. Because of how well we get on I trust her and am open to anything she wants to try. She is never less than hugely positive, which is one of the most important qualities in someone, as far as I am concerned. After meeting Nichola it is fair to say this stopped being a diet and became a lifestyle and what a wonderful one it is.

That's one of the best pieces of advice I can give someone who wants to lose a lot of weight, surround yourself with positive people who will only support and encourage you. Beware of the naysayers, you will have enough of a battle on your hands with your own hunger pangs, or whatever, you do not need to put up with someone else's bad attitude on top of that.

Today, my relationship with food is a far healthier one. I can appreciate that something smells and looks delicious, but I don't feel the need to have a plate of it. Sometimes just a chip or a spoonful of Shelly's dinner will be enough to sooth the desire to eat something taboo. Thanks to Nicola I know what suits my body and what doesn't, so it is easy to stay away from certain foods because I have the knowledge. It is just plain common sense to avoid stuff that will make me feel crap. I suppose I'm lucky in that I really like good food, for instance I love fruit and use it in the way that someone else might use sweets. On a summer's day I will make ice lollies from cordial instead of buying an ice-cream-based ice-pop.

For the first time in my life I have known what it is to feel healthy I won't eat anything that will jeopardise that. I do, from time to time, enjoy something like a nice meal, but only on special occasions and for the moment that's the way it will stay until I reach my goal. I would never give up this feeling of health for any food as it really does feel better than any food and it lasts a lot longer too.

My diet is simple, 70 per cent is vegetables and 30 per cent is made up of fish or meat or poultry. Initially I did wonder how I was going to eat so many vegetables but then, like everything else, I got used to it. The only problem is the price of keeping the fridge full of fresh produce, but that's another story. I don't worry about eating out in restaurants as it is easy to order a meal that fits perfectly into my diet, which is the great thing about keeping it simple. To be honest, I dislike referring to it as a 'diet' because that implies it is a temporary situation and I will go back to eating everything else, at some stage, something I have no intention of doing. As far as I am concerned I have found a 'diet' for life, balanced and leaving me full – not bloated and lethargic – at the end of every meal; this is my lifestyle.

A TYPICAL DAY

6am: Wake up to warm water with the juice from half a lemon

6.30–8.30am: Training

8:30am: Fish (hake) with apple cider vinegar or a spinach omelette or Greek yoghurt with mixed seeds

11pm: protein drink

1pm: fish or turkey mince or red meat with vegetables, e.g.: spinach, broccoli, cauliflower, mushrooms, leeks, celery, peppers, chillies, beetroot, lettuce/salad leaves, raw carrot, red onions; or omelette with side salad

If I am in college I will eat cold chicken or fish with salad

3pm: protein drink or Greek yoghurt with mixed seeds

5:30pm: training

7pm: fish or turkey mince or red meat with vegetables, as above

Note: Also I can eat fruit, if I want to. I particularly enjoy mixed berries with a few almonds which slows down the release of sugar, or else I would have a red apple or a few grapes.

In April I got to run my first 5k with the *Ray D'Arcy Show*'s 'Join Spar and Ray for 5k' in Limerick, I had trained very well for it. Running, for me, is a really enjoyable experience; for so long I struggled to walk so running is an amazing feeling of freedom for me. I was surprised when the show asked me to be the special guest starter for the race and I was proud to accept, especially as it was in Limerick. On the day I was accompanied by a friend of mine, Angela, who I met at the Dublin Marathon and who ran the 5k course with me. I completed the run in forty-six minutes and it was a very special day for me as it was a massive difference to the previous year's 5ks in Dublin and Cork. I felt an amazing sense of pride in my accomplishment. Just a few days later, I did it again at the Join Spar and Ray for 5k in the Phoenix Park, Dublin; this time I got to run with a very special group of friends from all around the country who became friends through Facebook, it really was a wonderful day in great company.

In May I took part in my second marathon, the Great Limerick Run. I would love to be able to write that it was physically a whole lot easier than my first one, but that would be a complete and utter lie! Although perhaps I should point out that it took place a mere four days before my end of year exams, and anyone who has ever done an exam will surely agree that it is a stressful time without doing a marathon on top of it. Fortunately I had great help in the form of Shelly, who kept me supplied with water and encouragement, and our friend Denyse, who had decided to run her first marathon after meeting me and who has become a good friend. We set a pace of walking 5k an hour, breaking the monotony with a 50m jog, every now and then, thus increasing our pace. There was a great atmosphere, despite the fact the number of competitors was smaller than expected, it was still a great crowd, to say nothing of the spectators.

Everything was going well until we hit the 10k mark, when I started to experience a vague sort of discomfort in my bowels and stomach. Assuming it was just gas I didn't pay much attention, expecting it to pass, but it didn't. By 15k, the half-way mark, the discomfort had turned into painful cramps and I made for the first bathroom I could see, believing that a quick shedding of the contents of my bowels was all that was required. Sadly this was not the case and the pain continued as I got back on route. I didn't know what else to do except to keep putting one foot in front of another. It was time to eat; I had had an early breakfast at 6am, two hours before the race began, but how could I put food into my painful belly, wouldn't it only make it worse? So, I went without, instead just sticking to water, hoping that it would do the trick of easing the pain. Only it didn't.

The pain got worse, zapping my energy level. As soon as I spied one of the portaloo cabins, I went inside, feeling drunk from exhaustion and something else. It was scary not knowing why this was happening and whether I should give into it or not. I sat there and, am not ashamed to admit, cried for maybe fifteen minutes, convinced that I wasn't going to be able to continue.

Don't ask me how, but I managed to do just that. I gathered myself together, closed the door of the cabin – my temporary sanctuary – behind me, to re-join Denyse and face into the toughest part of the course, while doing my best to shake off the feeling that I was slightly out of it. Shelly came to meet us, something which remains a blur to me, and she was immediately worried on seeing how emotional and pale I was.

At 25k I felt a bit better, emotionally and mentally at least. I was still too afraid to eat, but Shelly made sure I had plenty of water. Physically I was wiped and it had become necessary to stop every couple of kilometres to rest for ten minutes or so until I found the strength to get moving again. As we headed back towards the city I had expected to get a mental boost, just like at the Dublin City Marathon, when Chris and I turned towards the city centre, but no such luck. All I could think about was that we had to go into the city before heading back out for the 10k route. Also, we were now making our way through the crowd of runners, who had completed the race, and their family and friends, who were headed home. In other words we were besieged with delighted well-wishers who asked us how we got on, leaving Denyse and I to explain that we were still in the middle of it, which we could well have done without thinking about at that point.

Just over Sarsfield Bridge, Mam and Nicole were waiting to cheer me on. Afterwards Mam told me she got an awful fright when she saw how white I was. In truth I was in agony by now and while I could cope with the pain, I was freaked by my sheer lack of energy and was starting to experiencing dizzy spells that forced me to sit down until they passed. As we walked very, very slowly, by Thomond Park, Rob, my brother, appeared, offering to walk with us, but I said no. I needed every ounce of concentration I had to keep going at this dead, slow pace. In my head I was literally repeating the words 'Left, right, left, right' over and over again. I knew I would finish the race, but that was about all I knew.

There was no official finishing line by the time Denyse and I reached it, only the line formed by family and friends, which was better than any official line. Unfortunately we were too late for medals, but still we had done it – we finished the Great Limerick Run in ten hours and thirty minutes, and not a moment too soon. I am not ashamed to say that without Shelly and Denyse I would have probably called it a day, but it is amazing what women nagging will make you do!

The best thing about it, perhaps, was the fact that apart from feeling stiff I suffered no crash, nor damaged feet, as I had after the Dublin run. The following morning there were no blisters and the stiffness improved with my hour's swim, which was a massive improvement on last's year marathon. Great, so I just had the exams to worry about now!

Saturday, 3 June was an extremely special day to me as this was the day I achieved another of my goals: the Try Athy, my first triathlon, comprising of a 1,500 metre swim, immediately followed by a 40km cycle and, lastly, a 10km run/walk. This was a test on many levels. Chris was doing it with me, with the plan being that we would start on our own, fifteen minutes ahead of the first wave of competitors. I hadn't done much cycling in ten years or so, in fact I only got on a bike for the first time in ten years just two days before Athy, but I was really looking forward to every section of the event, anxious to see how I would do in a triathlon where my weight wouldn't be a factor with the first two sections, swimming and cycling, so I could almost believe that I had as good a chance as any of the others of finishing. It wasn't just the actual sports themselves that had to be performed; there was also the two transitions, the first taking place between the river swim and the cycle, which involved stripping out of my wetsuit in front of the town square. The thought of this part alone had terrorised me somewhat but then, on the actual day, I didn't give a second thought as to who could see my body or not. In the end, all that mattered was changing and jumping onto my bike, fully kitted out, as fast as I could.

I ran out of drinking water, a rookie mistake, about kilometre from the end of the cycling route. Also, I was not prepared for aching shoulders and hands from gripping the handle bars. A sore bum I expected, however, and this I definitely had. I have to say that I received great support from my fellow competitors, as throughout the different parts of the race someone would wish me well or tell me to keep going and that I was doing great.

The transition from the bike back to the ground was a tough one. I was sluggish at this point, my poor legs felt like I had lead in my runners, but I figured they would loosen up after a bit, allowing me to run properly. As competitors passed me by they yelled at me to hang in there. The sense of camaraderie was more important to me than winning a gold medal. As we hit the half-way mark of the running section, 5k, we were the last athletes on the path though we met the rest on their way back to the finish line, which was behind us. Again, I was encouraged to keep going and that I was almost there.

Unfortunately my legs could not recover enough, after the hard cycle, to allow me to run at all but I really didn't mind, I was just delighted to be taking part in my first triathlon. Although I did hope that I might be able to run the last few hundred metres. Chris and I counted down the kilometres we had left to walk – four, three, two, one – trying to stick to a time average of thirteen minutes per kilometre. My legs groaned but I just kept doing what I always do, at a time like this, put one foot in front of the other.

As we turned into the last five hundred metres, we spied, in the distance, the flags marking the finish line, along with Shelly and Carly, a welcome sight indeed. We walked another 300 metres or so before I said to Chris, 'Come on!' and broke into a run. This was to be the very first time that I would cross a proper finish line at a big event and I was determined to do it as best I could.

This event stands out as one of my proudest achievements to date. It took us approximately five hours and twenty-five minutes to complete the course, broken down as follows: 1,500m swim – 47:53; 40km cycle – 2:19:01; 10km run – 2:09:46. I'll be honest, while I was very happy with my swim time and happy enough with the cycling; I was disappointed with the running. However it just gives me something to improve on for the next triathlon.

CHAPTER EIGHT

DUBLIN CITY MARATHON 2012

Bank Holiday Monday, 29 October 2012: the morning of the 33rd Dublin City Marathon (DCM), and my second time as a competitor.

A few days beforehand I had been on the *Ray D'Arcy Show* and he told me that the *Irish Times* journalist, Roisín Ingle, who was doing the marathon for the first time, had decided that she was going to start her race at 6am, three hours before the official starting time. I don't know if she had heard about my experience from the 2011 event, trying to find road signs, and finishing in the dark at 8pm, long after the finish line had been dismantled and the majority of supporters and competitors had gone home.

On hearing this, my first reaction was, no way, that's not for me! I wanted to be at that start line and be part of that very special atmosphere. However, as I thought about it a bit more, it began to seem like a brilliant idea and much safer than last year.

Now, don't get me wrong. I absolutely loved my marathon experience last year. It was a huge turning point for me to have taken part and completed the course – despite the late hour and the comparative silence that greeted Chris and me as we finally crossed the finish line. At the same time I could not forget the 'loneliness', for the want of a better word. For most of the race it was just Chris and me, we got lost and poor Ray D'Arcy and Jenny had to get into their car, on a wet, winter's evening and come find us.

It was also unnerving, as well as potentially dangerous; negotiating the heavy Bank Holiday traffic, in the dark, after the roads had been opened up again, trying to cross busy streets for a race that had long finished for everyone else. This year I was hoping and hoping it would be different: I'd be with the other athletes I admired so much, and there would be plenty of rousing support.

Roisín's idea made perfect sense! I told Chris and he said he'd do whatever I wanted to do. So I contacted the race officials and got permission for the two of us to start our race at 6am.

Just like last year Chris and I were sharing a hotel room, not far from the starting line. After checking into the Mont Clare Hotel, we went out, like last year, for dinner with Emlyn from TriFit and his runner mates. Our wives were driving up from Limerick in the morning to check in and then come meet us at the finish line, about lunch-time.

We were back early enough from the restaurant. Lights out was 11pm sharp, no television! It was a typical night for me. I never sleep well before a race, constantly waking up throughout, but I don't get upset over it. As far as I'm concerned the sleepless night is all part and package of the buzz of the whole adventure.

Our alarms rang out at 4.30am. Last year we made the time to enjoy a leisurely hotel breakfast, this year we were way too early for one so I made do with a banana. In any case, with the day ahead, my excitement ensured that I had little or no appetite so the banana went down easily and quickly.

Breakfast over, I packed my knapsack, making sure I included my rain jacket, water, plasters, food, Deep Heat and talcum powder. The food was the same as last year, health food Chia Bia bars and more bananas.

It was 5.40am when we left the hotel, walking out into a cold, dark morning, and making our way to the start line. I was extremely glad for my hat and gloves as the air was more than chilly. I was and I wasn't nervous. I mean, I knew I could definitely do it, because this was my third marathon. Furthermore I knew I had trained hard for it so I knew I would improve on last year's performance. But no matter how confident I was in my ability, it was a still an actual marathon and so not to be underestimated as they are very hard – so it wasn't going to be an easy day, either way.

Okay. So we were starting early in order to enjoy, and benefit from, the experience of having people around us later on in the day. To have that support later on in the race, we had had to give up on having people around us at the starting line. Therefore, there was hardly anyone around at 6am, save for a few race officials who looked at us in vague confusion, as if to say, *Er, what are you doing here? It doesn't start for another three hours.*

To say it was quiet and lacking in atmosphere would be an understatement. I had thrived on the energy from the crowds of runners and supporters last year as I stood waiting to start my race. Nevertheless I knew I'd have both of them, in spades, within a few short hours.

I'm trying to remember how I felt, what was going through my head. Was this marathon more important to me than last year's? To be honest, I couldn't and still wouldn't choose between the two of them. 2012 was my first DCM and it will always hold a very special place in my heart. Last year I was 29 stone 5lbs. This year I was I was 25 stone 4lbs and hoping to improve on that first performance, thereby seeing, for myself, how much I had improved in my training and confidence. Every marathon, I would imagine, whether it's their first or tenth, is as special to any runner or walker, like me.

Using my phone to time ourselves, we started bang on at 6am, taking a photograph as proof. We took off a good, strong pace and it wasn't long before I was peeling off my gloves and hat. As I warmed up, I started to relax more. There was an undeniable peacefulness to the city, as we strode through its centre at this hour on a Bank Holiday morning. I was having trouble believing that the empty streets would be crawling with people in another little while.

There didn't seem to be any signs up yet to direct the runners, not that Chris and I could see and, as a result, we found ourselves slightly lost over by the Rotunda Hospital. A friendly taxi driver, who was waiting for the lights to change, told us that we should have taken a left instead of walking straight ahead. We thanked him and retraced our steps. This wouldn't be the last time we would become confused about where we were meant to go!

In no time at all we reached the Phoenix Park and promptly got lost again. I had to smile. It was now about 8am and the park was deserted, or, at least, it appeared to be. There was still little or no signage, and we turned right when we should have turned left, ending up at an exit some distance away from where we should have been. Once again we had to double back on ourselves, taking a new road that was adjacent to the perimeter, which we hoped would bring us back to the Chapelizod exit.

Eventually I recognised where we were, having ran this route a few months earlier for the 'Join Ray for 5K'. We both felt a lot happier now that we knew where we were and where we were to go. Being unsure of the route is a big distraction; it was time to start focusing on our pace again. However, now a second distraction made its appearance, in the form of a bloody massive – albeit beautiful – stag standing a mere thirty feet away from us and looking ready for something.

This was Chris' first sighting of a deer and he faltered, wondering loudly if we should turn back. I'm not sure if I can admit to being as nervous as Chris. In my mind it came down to this: getting lost twice had eaten into our self-allotted time so I wasn't prepared to lose any more minutes. I refused to consider any alternative to making loud noises which, thankfully, sent the stag trotting away from us. A mighty relief, until, that is, there was a clumsy shuffle in the bushes beside us, and we spied an even bigger pair of antlers, peeping out at us. This, unsurprisingly, boosted our speed all the way up the hill. From here, at a safe distance, we enjoyed the sight of a large herd of deer to our left, in the morning sunshine. It was breath-taking.

Soon after, we found the right exit and the first real signs of life. Officials were stocking up one of the water stations that would be fuelling over 14,000 runners in another hour or so. As we continued along, members of the public started to take their spots at the side of the road, to be in plenty of time to cheer on their friends and relatives.

We were both pleased with how we were doing. My goal had been to be half-way done by 10am and this is more or less where we were, on the Crumlin Road, knowing it would be a matter of minutes until we saw the elite runners. The weather was perfect, mild without wind or rain. If you remember, last year Chris and I competed most of the race in wet clothes through the depressing sheets of rain.

About 1,000 metres from the halfway point Chris and I were momentarily enveloped by the 'elite' group. These were the 'real' runners, the twenty or thirty professionals – Kenyans, other Africans, Europeans, including some Irish – who were all muscle and determination to win every marathon they participate in. In other words, they were like the 'A-Listers' of Hollywood movie stars. They are hard-core athletes, who train and run to win. It was marvellous to watch them sail by us with enviable ease and grace.

I loved their grace – they really are amazing – but they make running at such a fast pace look so easy you can't help but think, 'Feck them for making it look so easy!'

At this point the roads were closed to traffic. Chris and I did our absolute best to stay to one side of the road, so as not to be in any runner's way. When we rounded a corner we went wide as the runners always went tight, staying as close as possible to the kerb. When it was necessary we took to the path, so determined was I not to ruin someone else's chances by getting in their way and slowing them down; I believe it's just good manners also.

A steady stream of runners passed us by, still allowing us breathing room on the road itself. Then, by mile fifteen, which brought me by my publishers, The O'Brien Press, in Rathgar, it got very busy indeed. Chris and I made for the path, which proved to be great fun as we were in with the cheery supporters.

It occurred to me that I was really doing very well. At this point, last year, I was in agony, having to stop every few minutes to stretch. This year my pace was still steady and I was thoroughly enjoying myself. Obliged to walk in single file, because the path was so busy, I was free to walk on in silence, and reflect on how well my body was coping.

Three miles later I started to feel a bit sore. In all fairness we had now been walking for six hours, but I was still enjoying myself and savouring the atmosphere of the crowds of runners some of whom yelled out their encouragement to me, and the onlookers who clapped and cheered on all the competitors, that couldn't but spur me on. This was what I had wanted from the day, to feel like I was a valuable part of the 'team'.

Someone tapped me on the shoulder. It was Sharon Ashmore, a friend from Leixlip. She asked me for a kiss as she whizzed by. Next we met Emlyn and his wife Vicky, from TriFit, who stopped to say to a quick hello before taking off again. There is something very special about meeting up with people you know, in the midst of a huge crowd, when you are undertaking something tough like a marathon. Just as last year, when my parents and Nicole came out to meet me, I found my emotions being stirred up and had to fight back the tears.

Along the way people lined both sides of the streets, handing out jellies to anyone who was in need of a sugar rush. Some of them were waving hand-made signs, willing the competitors to keep going. I found it oddly moving. The spectators just looked so bloody happy, for themselves and for us, as they provided a constant supply of support, calling out stuff like, 'Go on! You can do it! Well done!' I suppose, looking back on last year, I had only a brief encounter with this sort of thing because Chris and I found ourselves so quickly left behind by the rest of the runners. Today was a much more positive experience thanks to our 6am start.

At one point, a little girl of no more than three or four years of age approached me and Chris, asking if we'd like a jelly. I wanted to weep with something; I'm not sure what, gratitude or maybe just the sheer joy of being there. A few minutes later the lads from the Irish Air Corps ran by in perfect formation.

At mile nineteen we reached 'Heartbreak Hill', or Roebuck Hill, just at the junction with Foster Avenue. It is a steep hill, the biggest on the route, and is approximately seven kilometres from the finish line, and because of that it is a bit of a killer. To have to run or walk uphill so far into the race is a tough one, whichever way you look at it. Also it's a long, gradual climb so you are waiting for what seems like ages before you head downhill again.

Fortunately, however, there are always a generous number of people who stand there to cheer the runners on, recognising that it is a difficult spot. It was here that we met Ray. He surprised me by saying I looked terrible. Obviously I felt better than I looked. In fact I was feeling quite sore now, along with experiencing the odd cramp in my legs, but it was nothing compared to the absolute hell I was in this time last year. It was just a brief chat with Ray before we walked on again.

On and on and on.

I had plenty of time to think about things. I'm sure the reader will realise by now that I tend to analyse, to the nth degree, my life and self. When you are walking constantly for eight or nine hours, at a stretch, you sure have a lot of time to reflect on life, the universe and such things. In any case I found myself reflecting on the last twelve months, since October 2011. Being perfectly honest, regarding my weight loss I wasn't exactly over the moon with just being over five stone lighter since the last DCM. Yet, I can't continually find fault with me without making sure I also appreciated the good stuff. It isn't fair if you don't, sometimes, at least, remember to pat yourself on the back too.

And what I had got to appreciate? Well, I had a newfound sense of belief in myself. It has been an uphill climb and I'm still climbing, but I'm moving on from the past. Every footstep I was taking along the route of this marathon was so much more than that for me. Most of my fellow runners would probably have shared this feeling of doing something important, if only for themselves. Maybe that's what makes a marathon so special. It's bloody hard but if you just keep moving, whichever way suits you best, you'll do it just fine.

Unlike last year, as Chris and I turned onto the Stillorgan Road, starting to head back towards the city, we were still amongst the hundreds of other runners. It was a far cry from stumbling along in the dark, hoping against hope we were – literally – on the right track. Most of the people around us didn't look too happy. We were all finding it tough now, all fighting our own personal battles. I did worry somewhat about people disagreeing with me starting so early but, then again, all I had received, and was still receiving, from the others, was pure goodwill, wishing me on to the finish line.

As we neared the city centre the crowd of tired competitors began to thin out. There were still plenty of people, but nowhere near the same volume as earlier. There were more friendly faces, but also a lot more pain. There were some who had picked up injuries, cramped legs or battered feet. There were those who had clearly hit the wall, but refused to stop. The agony was stretched across their pale, drawn faces but still, like Derek Redmond, they kept going.

Coming towards Ballsbridge my own wall was meeting me. My energy was just about spent and I was sore all over, except for my feet, for which I was hugely grateful. Nevertheless I was still happy and, hand on heart, still enjoying myself.

At mile twenty-four I became mindful of the time. If I dug deep enough we could come in under eight hours and forty-six minutes. There was the perfect motivation to quicken my pace. However, my legs did not seem to be communicating with my brain or maybe it was the other way around. All I could do was hope that I was walking a bit faster than I had been. It was honestly hard to judge at the stage.

With about a mile and a half to go we caught up with a guy who looked to be in some trouble. He was a runner who was now just about walking along, though it was more like limping. Of course I knew exactly what he was going through so I couldn't just ignore him. Chris and I slowed down to ask him if he was okay and then, between us, we kept him chatting, just as Ray and the others had done for us last year, to distract from the distance that persisted between us and the finish line. We tried to get him to pick up his pace so that we could keep him with us. The fact of the matter is, rightly or wrongly, time was very important to me now and, yes, we did make to leave him behind, as he was unable to move his legs any faster, but my conscience prevented me from careering ahead so we slowed down again. I could not have left him by himself, I just couldn't have. Fortunately, just before mile twenty-five, he was joined by a friend of his and we were happy enough to say goodbye.

As we approached the turn that would bring us around by Trinity College the streets were lined with ecstatic spectators and delighted runners. I could understand the pain of my fellow runners, having experienced it first-hand myself, but I also fully understood the pride in their faces. My God! We were almost bloody there. Coming up the side of the Davenport Hotel Chris and I had our first sighting of our beautiful wives, who were madly waving at us. Beside them were our friends Angela and Wayne, cheering and clapping. We also could see the finish line before turning right for the last loop.

I didn't care about that last loop, which may sound brazen or flippant, but at mile twenty-five I knew I was almost there and that was all I could think about ...I was almost there. At that point I thought of this great quote that I had found, which best explains my state of mind, and every line is true:

At Mile 20 I thought I was dead

At Mile 22 I wished I was dead

At Mile 24 I knew I was dead

At Mile 26.2 I realised ... I had become too tough to kill.

To be honest that last bit, the walking around Trinity College, is a bit of a blur. I wish I had more details for you but honestly I was just so, so tired by then. There were cheering crowds and runners willing themselves on to the end, using every last bit of strength they could muster from within, which was exactly what I was concentrating on. So, I can't remember who was behind or in front of me. I don't think I even glanced at the spectators, at this point. It was all about my continuing to put one foot in front of the other. The sun was shining, I think. And that's pretty much all I can remember.

Completing the lap around Trinity we turned for the final home stretch of maybe four hundred metres or so. Barriers were needed here because there were so many people pressing forward, to see their loved ones cross that beautiful finish line. What a rush! Chris and I pressed forward, carried on by the atmosphere and the sheer ecstasy of having done it, once again. Whatever you might think about us starting three hours before anyone else I can only offer you my genuine gratitude, for a bloke like me to be able to finish a marathon while the line was intact, with race officials, fellow runners and cheering crowds. It's my only defence and explanation. I just hope that any naysayers out there cannot doubt the importance, for me, to finish the race while it's still in session. There were no short cuts, I did the same route as everyone else – even an extra piece – it's just that I really wanted, as much as possible, to do it *with* everyone for no other reason than that I look up to and admire them so very much.

We crossed the line at 2.48pm, having taken eight hours and forty-eight minutes to complete the course. In other words we had knocked one hour and fifty-eight minutes of our previous time. I was absolutely beside myself with joy. Chris and I did our manly-guy thing and shook hands in triumph but then, when Chris could plainly see the emotion in my face, he gave me a hug. Neither of us said a word. We just kept walking.

The tears flowed down my face and I was too tired to do anything about them. My heart was just bursting with pride, relief and joy. I know I've used the word a few times now but I honestly can't think of another one. Joy! I had now completed three marathons, two triathlons and a half marathon. Over fifteen stone separated me from the guy who couldn't have walked from the couch to the kitchen without stopping to catch my breath, the infertile guy who was now going to be a father within a few short months. It all just hit me in those few moments of stepping across that line. All this change, all the pain, all the fear and anxiety, had been worth it. Yes, there are people who might think, *What's all the fuss? It's just a marathon.* However, it was so much more than that to me.

After we collected our medals Chris and I met the girls and headed for the hotel. On the way we passed a guy in a wheelchair. He was just beginning his final lap and his face said it all. His wheelchair wasn't a special type of wheelchair adapted for marathons. No, it was just an ordinary one that he had had to roll for twenty-six miles. He stopped me in my tracks. I felt humbled and privileged to be able to take part in an event with someone like him. For me, this is the marathon: fifteen thousand athletes with fifteen thousand stories as to why they are there, pushing themselves to do something excruciatingly painful, just to be able to say, like me, that they had done it. They had actually gone and bloody well done it.

It may sound profound, but for me events like this are never about adulation, finish lines or medals. I spent my life looking at such events and at the athletes I admire so much, thinking 'I could never do anything like that!', so by doing it I am proving to myself that I *can* do the things I never thought possible. This has given me a huge sense of what I am capable of and has made me a much stronger and more resilient person; I know if I keep going I can finish this. If I can do this, doesn't it mean that I can do anything else I put my mind to?

People sometimes tell me that I train an awful lot, but I explain to them that a guy of my size, who wants to be able to do marathons, has to. Normal training for an average-size guy just isn't adequate when I know that my marathon is going to involve between eight and ten hours walking, longer than most people's working day, and my body has to be able to endure that. I swim five mornings a week and I am sure that my diary makes it obvious how much I enjoy this. Honestly, I cannot emphasise this enough, swimming is a great way to start the day and utterly therapeutic, both mentally and physically. About five evenings a week I'm in the gym with Chris, working on my strength and conditioning. I also like to get two walks in midweek, while on Sundays I do a big walk, lasting maybe four or five hours. All this walking is necessary, to toughen up my legs and feet so that they won't cause me trouble during an event. Recently I have added cycling to my regime, as I mean to do many more triathlon events.

Sport has become very important to me for all the reasons that I've presented throughout. What I personally like about setting sports-based goals is that they are, unlike other types of ambitions, actually attainable if you only practise hard enough, unless, of course, you dream of playing in the FA Cup final and score the winning goal in the ninetieth minute. Seriously, though, there is such a variety of sports to choose from, catering for all tastes. If like me, your weight narrowed down your life to a worn spouse and blood relatives, joining a team, be it basketball, football or running, instantly improves your social life. For some, that may sound like a big jump too soon, so you could do what I did, swim alone and work out at home until you feel confident enough to join a class. If you struggle with depression or dark moods that swamp you for days on end, try breaking the pattern with exercise. It's not just about physically feeling better; it's also about a positive mindset, which is definitely required when dieting and setting out on the road to better health and fitness. Plus the more positive you feel, the more confident you are. It's a win-win situation, as far as I'm concerned.

Some people may not see the merits of me doing such events, but I do them for me, not for a medal, but to prove to myself that I can. I admire sports people so much especially runners, triathletes and crossfitters, for me it is an absolute privilege to be at events with people I admire. I'm so fortunate that, for the most part, I am warmly accepted. These events aren't for everybody, but for me the marathons, 5ks and triathlons have proved to be some of the best days of my life because I tested myself, I did something I only ever dreamed of and, more importantly, I didn't give up. Much like my mantra, 'If I do not give up I cannot fail', I finished the races and enjoyed the feelings of accomplishment. These are the stepping stones that keep me going on this very long journey.

And for anyone who is reading this, and knows someone who is trying to lose weight can I suggest that you don't constantly ask them how it is going. I can tell you exactly how it is going, and that is *tough*! Only, it doesn't help to talk about that, about the fact that it is hard and that there are days when you break the diet out of hunger or because you just felt too bad not to, and then you are hit by a guilt so heavy, you have to reason with yourself that you haven't actually committed murder or beaten up an old-aged pensioner. Just tell them they look great! Believe me, you have no idea how powerful those three words are to someone like me.

CHAPTER NINE

SHELLY'S STORY

When I started thinking about doing this book and what shape I hoped it would take, there was one thing I had decided on, from the very beginning. I gave my version of the story, as best I could, but it would be unfair to leave it just at that. One of the reasons I am doing the book is that I genuinely hope it will help someone out there. Therefore, it was always my plan to give Shelly an opportunity to tell her side of the story. Perhaps there is somebody out there reading this book, right now, who is feeling unable to make the big decision to change. And, maybe what I have described, from my own personal experience isn't – for the want of a better word – dramatic enough. Without sounding preachy, it is important to realise that your happiness or unhappiness with yourself has a direct effect on those who love you.

* * *

SHELLY'S STORY:

The first time I saw Gary, I was on a night out with my mates, in one of the local bars here in Limerick. He was sitting at a nearby table and I couldn't help noticing his lovely smile, as he joked around with his friends. I turned to my friend and said, 'He's really cute!' I didn't approach him or anything; I'm much too shy for that. He was well built – I've never found thin guys attractive – and handsome. His smile is definitely one of my favourite things about him.

At the time I was working as a store detective for Brown Thomas and, shortly after that, we found ourselves working for the same security firm, and struck up a jokey, flirtatious friendship. I think one of my friends had to tell him that I liked him, I certainly would never have told him. Eventually, we kissed and dated for a short while.

We broke up because he felt I was getting too serious and he didn't feel ready to commit to anything longterm. I was upset but he was younger than me so I tried to be realistic in my mind about it. He doesn't know it but after we parted, and I had changed jobs, I talked about him to anyone who would listen. I moved home to my parents' house in Tipperary and commuted to Limerick after I got a job working two nights a week in one of the nightclubs. One night I was in the club, it was early yet so it wasn't that busy, so you couldn't miss any of the new arrivals. Gary walked in with a group of friends and my heart jumped. I told my colleague, who was standing beside me, as casually as I could, 'Oh, there's my ex.'

The nightclub had two floors so I was frequently on the move between them, when we finally 'bumped' into one another on the stairs. I may have had something to do with that! Anyway I said a quick, 'Hi!', as did he and continued on my way, as did he. But something stopped us. We turned around at the exact same time and walked back to one another, started talking properly and then exchanged our new phone numbers.

After my shift finished I drove home to Tipperary. He sent me a text that very same evening, actually it was more like 4am, to which I gladly replied, and we continued texting for ages after. So we started going out again and this time it felt different. I just knew that it was meant to be, especially after he left a message on my phone, one night, when the battery had died. I recharged it and saw that I had missed several calls from him, and then I listened to his message in which he said he was worried because he couldn't reach me and hoped that I was okay. Suddenly he said those words that made me breathe a sigh of relief, although I wasn't expecting to hear them so soon; he told me he loved me. I could tell he didn't mean to say them, he sounded slightly aghast that he had said them aloud, but my heart nearly exploded and I rang him back immediately.

We had a wonderful wedding, even if I say so myself. I've never been into weddings, unlike some of my friends, and relied heavily, on Orla, Gary's sister to help me put one together. Our wedding was the first full wedding I have ever been to, having only ever been invited to the 'afters' part. One of the reasons I loved the day so much was that, with one exception, we had all our nieces and nephews around us, and if there was one thing Gary and I had in common, it was that we were both mad about kids.

He needed to have his wedding suit made, at the very last minute, but that didn't bother me. I never thought to myself, 'Oh, Jesus! He needs to lose weight!' All I cared about was that he felt comfortable in himself. When others ribbed him about losing weight I would become very defensive and protective of his feelings. Anyway, I thought he looked smashing on the day, if a bit pale beside me and my fake tan. He bought a cheap pair of wedding shoes in Dunnes Stores so we had made sure to bring a pair of runners in which he could change into when the new ones started to hurt. He put them on as soon as we reached the hotel. A few of the guests were telling him to leave on the shoes, to keep the look, until after the meal, but I said no, leave him alone; he's fine as he is. It was our day after all.

The honeymoon was not without its difficulties. On the plane over I know it killed him that I had to spend the long flight squashed and half twisted around so that we could fit into the seat together. It would be years before he'd get on a plane again. I wish now that we could have just stayed in Las Vegas, where he was happier, although we didn't do as much touring as I would have liked because the heat was affecting him so much. He became a bit of a recluse in Cancun, preferring to stay in the hotel room. I accepted this, I knew he didn't feel comfortable in the dining room and assumed it was to do with the narrowness of the chairs. However, it meant that I ate alone – on my honeymoon. The food was all-inclusive, with a full buffet provided, so I would fill my plate, sit down by myself, and eat it quickly before going back up to fill a plate for Gary. Worried that people were staring at me, thinking I was greedy, going up twice for two dinners, I would tell the staff as loudly as I could, for the other guests to hear, 'My husband is still feeling unwell. Could I have a tray to bring his dinner up to him?' Stupid, I know.

It is all such a blur now, regarding his weight. People, mostly his concerned family, would whisper to me that he was getting bigger and bigger, and needed to be careful for his health. I would never know how to respond to this and shied away from broaching it with him as I knew it would only worsen his mood. When things started going badly, when the business went bust and so on, he would go for ages without admitting to me that he was seriously worried about stuff. Then there would be a sudden out-pouring in one go, when he would blurt out every single thing that was bothering him, but he never, ever mentioned his weight as being one of them. So, how could I have heaped that onto him when he was so caught up worrying about money, the banks and our future?

We never mentioned it, the fact he was piling on weight. His only response was to go online and order clothes in a bigger size. In any case what could I say, because I was starting to pile on weight too? He did his best to encourage me to lose it and, before he grew too heavy, we would go out walking where I would struggle to keep up with his long stride. That might seem hypocritical that he wanted me to lose weight but it wasn't for him, he was reacting to how upset I got because I felt fat and unattractive. I'm sure most women recognise what I'm talking about, when you pull your wardrobe apart to find something that makes you feel good. We stopped going out for meals or drinks because I got so stressed trying to find something decent to wear. Then it became the both of us worrying about our clothes fitting us and how we looked. He stopped coming to Tipperary for my family stuff and I made excuse after excuse for him that usually involved blaming the dog needing to be minded.

Things got very bad after we both lost our jobs in 2009. Lots of people, I'm sure, were going through a little of what we were experiencing, sending out one job application after another, never knowing if it had been received or not. The pressure of debts and bills weighed heavily on us and, if I hadn't had to walk the dog, I might have just stayed in the house too, like Gary. Food, I think, became his way of coping with everything. He had zero interest in going outside and this is when the weight really crept up on him. I had to do everything, while he took to the couch, watching me put skirting boards on the walls because his knees could no longer bear his weight for more than a few minutes at a time. When I was finished I had to go and make his cup of tea, for the same reason.

I loved him throughout, but it did get hard. I felt like I had become, without realising it, a carer instead of a wife. The only time I had to myself was when I took the dog out for a walk, and that became increasingly precious to me.

When I visited my parents Gary would ring me to see when I was coming home, not out of control, but because he genuinely needed my help every single day. I worried that I wasn't helping him, mentally, as I should but I honestly didn't know any better, I put up with his mood swings and did my best not to upset him. I just wanted 'my' Gary back, the smiling, handsome guy I had fallen in love with, and I had to believe that he was still there somewhere, beneath the anger and depression or else what was the point.

We did go to Weightwatchers for a while, but I was the only one who lost weight, which was frustrating for him. The same thing happened with the Lipotrim diet. I lost three stone in nine weeks while he just caught one chest infection after another.

I began to worry about him all the time. When I went out I would become afraid that he would die in my absence, not so much from suicide as from a heart attack. The irony is that I knew I didn't have to fret about him killing himself since I knew he was very worried about how his dead body would be removed from the house and the fact there mightn't be a big enough coffin to bury him in. Nights were tortuous for me as he suffered from sleep apnoea, so if he was lying on his back he would frequently stop breathing for a few seconds until I nudged him to take a breath. It was impossible for me to sleep after that so we ended up in separate rooms. I obsessed about him falling down the stairs, when I was out shopping, or perhaps tripping up in the garden shed and being unable to get upright by himself. What if I arrived home and found him lying on the ground, how could I lift him, how many people would it take to get him in an ambulance? I'm ashamed to admit that this was the sort of stuff that occupied my thoughts.

When he decided to lose weight I was sceptical about him doing it by himself. He was so big that I couldn't see a way back to normality. I was never so glad as when he told me he emailed the *Ray D'Arcy Show*, and, on top of that, then accepted the invitation to visit the studios. That was a huge surprise to me in itself. When they offered their help I knew immediately that he couldn't give up now, he would have to stick to a diet because of their interest and support. For this alone I am truly grateful to Ray and his team. They provided the motivation that spurred him on, and continue to do so today. Then there is the legend, Chris, his personal trainer. I just cannot thank all these people enough for, perhaps, saving my husband's life.

He surprised me again when he decided to follow in my footsteps and return to college. I kept thinking, when I sat in my own lecture hall, that Gary would never survive a day, with the size of the seats, but he went ahead and filled out the forms and has never looked back.

His weight loss has had a huge impact on our relationship. He had become so bitter and guarded, which wasn't part of who he was. Now, thanks to being on the radio he was forced to open up about his problems, having to admit to his weight, and how it had affected him and me. Also, nobody knew we had been struggling with trying to have a baby. But he opened up about that too and I think this openness allowed us to have a fresh start. Every one of his goals are genuine and each weigh-in is a step closer to his ideal – a fit and healthy guy who can walk into a shop and buy normal-sized clothes, that don't cost the earth or take up most of my washing-line.

Life is so much easier these days, and I have my handsome, sociable man back, and the one who knows how to make me laugh anytime, anywhere. And just so you know, I never stopped fancying him, no matter what.

It isn't easy living with someone who hates themselves because of their weight, and I feel for anyone who is going through what I did. I was asked, for the book, what advice I might give to the partners, spouses or family members and, really, all I can say is to love them no matter what. They are down because they are angry at themselves and you have to remember that. Do your best to be there, when they want to talk, or even just rant about stupid stuff. They need to know that you are there for them. Make them feel special, even if it means you have to make a fool out of yourself, or do something you normally wouldn't, just hang in there to help break through their dark mood and bring them out of themselves.

If you get frustrated, don't take it out on them. Yes, I know this sounds a lot easier than it is, but two wrongs don't make a right. Thank God I had the dog to take out, allowing me to go and pound the almighty crap out of the pavement when the tension at home got too much for me.

Lastly, be their number one fan. I remember going for a walk with Gary, just before he went on the radio. For obvious reasons, we went out after dark and, still, the cars were slowing down so that the drivers and passengers could have a good gawp at the big man. Of course, it would never have occurred to them to appreciate the physical pain he was going through, just to walk along beside me. He was experiencing chronic pain in his back and legs. I took a deep breath and said, as cheerfully as I could, 'Jesus! We are flying along!' and I kept making comments like that, doing my best to distract us from the insolent stares. My heart broke for Gary and I wanted to flip the bird at the onlookers, or throw something at them – not that I ever would – but it was so hard to see people look at my husband like that.

Believe me, you'll find the strength, if you love them, you'll do anything for them. I suppose you have to work at never losing hope that it will can and will be better.

SHELLY KIRWAN

CHAPTER TEN

'PURE JOY'

Last Friday Shelly and I decided to go through my wardrobe and get rid of stuff that no longer fit me. I tried on everything with the result that three quarters of my clothes are in bags waiting to go to the local charity shop. I suppose this is one of the big moments in any dieter's life, when their old clothes confirm what their eyes mightn't see in the mirror.

I tried on my wedding jacket. I was somewhere between thirty-two and thirty-four stone when we got married, nowhere near my heaviest, and the jacket, I am proud to say, was swimming on me. Next I tried on a t-shirt that I wore when Shelly and I started going out together, and I'll be honest it was tight, but it fit me. How wonderful is that, to be able to go back in time and meet the shape I was all those years ago. After that I put on a pair of jeans that I first wore when I was starting college, last year. They just about fit me when I bought them, let's say they were snug. By the end of the college year, this year, they were a bit loose, and then, last Friday, they were far too big for me to ever contemplate wearing them again.

You might be surprised that I haven't gone waltzing out to buy new clothes yet. Most of those clothes that I threw out were bought online and were expensive, so I made them last for as long as I could. Nevertheless I am looking forward to the day I will walk into a shop and buy whatever I want off the rails.

There are mirrors around the house now. In fact we have a big mirror just inside the front door, in which I study my reflection on a daily basis. It's not out of vanity, I assure you; rather it is more to do with my own fascination with what is happening. I see myself emerging from my body as the fat disappears. I notice the definition of my muscles in my upper torso, my arms, shoulders and chest. For months I have been looking at my legs and my feet. The change in them has been massive. Talk about enjoying the simple pleasures in life, I get a huge thrill out of wiggling my toes and noting how the skin ripples over the bones. This is something I had never seen before.

To date I have lost fifteen and a half stone. I weigh 359lbs, or twenty-five stone nine pounds. Therefore I am still about nine and a half stone from my goal. At some stage I am going to require surgery to remove the loose, sagging skin because, apart from the unsightliness, it will prevent me from losing more weight.

So I am still in progress regarding the weight loss, but this story had been more than simply about that; while at times it is very slow and very frustrating I am continually losing weight and feeling better about myself and reaping the rewards. At times the slow weight-loss does test my resolve, but my experiences to date prove to me that I just need to keep going and I will get to the day when I see myself in the mirror and am truly happy with the person in the mirror. Not just the body, but more importantly what is underneath. Friday the thirteenth, I have written elsewhere, is considered unlucky for some, but let me tell you about Friday 13 July 2011 in my house.

A couple of days beforehand Shelly had been very down, after finding out, on Facebook, that a friend of hers was pregnant, shortly after we had been informed that our scheduled date at the Fertility Clinic had been pushed back. It had been a while since I had seen her so upset and, feeling helpless, I suggested that she go home to Tipperary for a couple days. She returned on the Friday, meeting me outside the TriFit gym and I drove us both home.

It had been a great work out session and I had the evidence with me. For ages I had been telling Chris that he could promote the gym online, suggesting that we record a session and post it as a short film. So I sat down at my computer and began working on the recording of the class, trying to edit it into a proper advertisement, which was hard going since it kept crashing the computer. I think since going back to college I enjoy such projects as it involves marketing.

I was about three hours or so, into it, doing my best to remain patient against another crash when Shelly appeared beside me, asking me to look at something. It took me a second to realise it was a pregnancy test. 'Is that a pink line or am I seeing things?' There was a definite pink line, I nodded, gulped and asked, 'What does this mean?' There was a moment's silence before she replied, 'I'm going out to get more'. I waited and waited. She was probably only gone about fifteen minutes but it felt like an eternity to me. Finally she reappeared with a few tests, including those advanced ones that tell you how far along you are.

Again, we waited and waited, until one of those tests informed us that we were between one and two weeks pregnant.

We stared in shock at one another. I was afraid to react. Not so long ago I had been told I was infertile. Then we were told that this was the wrong diagnosis but we would need treatment, which had been put off by a few months. What was going on? We held one another, tears running down both our faces. I felt pure joy and pure terror at the exact same time. There had been no preparation for this, all our energy had gone into trying to get pregnant, what to do when we achieved that was something we had not considered.

Somebody, I can't remember who, had said that they'd bet we'd get pregnant naturally. I joked, 'If that happens, I'll be demanding a DNA test!' I was so sure we would not be able to get pregnant without the treatment.

When I was able to speak I said, 'Now, what do we do?' We decided to wait for a while and keep it to ourselves, just in case we were imagining things or something – it's funny we knew so much about fertility treatments and what they entailed, but we had never got past that and we didn't know what to do once we got pregnant.

Less than an hour later my mother and Nicole arrived on a surprise visit. Shelly and I were, by this stage, grinning wildly from ear to ear. The plan to keep it to ourselves was flung to the wayside as soon as Mam asked us what we were smiling about. She cried with joy.

The next morning Shelly did another test, to be sure, to be sure. We were still pregnant. A couple of days later I found myself in the Limerick branch of Next, buying a changing table and cot, there was a sale on, Shelly was at home and I didn't think twice about it.

Some time later, Shelly and I went onto Ray's show to announce that we were three months pregnant. I had spoken openly about the problems involved in trying to get pregnant and, therefore, was hugely excited about telling the listeners. It was a privilege to have our good news blessed by so many strangers. A couple of people texted in that, much to their surprise, they were crying for joy for two people they had never met.

Our baby is due in March 2013; a new beginning, and one that I hardly dared even dream about.

EPILOGUE

When I see a very large person on the street the first thing I notice are elements of my old self – how they stare at the ground, avoiding eye contact, their posture demonstrating a lack of confidence and general unhappiness with themselves. To be honest I see myself, the person I used to be. But then I move past their figure to the person they are, because, well, you have to. It might be easier for me to do this, of course, since I have been there, and, in fact, am still there, judging from some of the looks that I get even now, though nowhere near as frequently as I used to. Perhaps just keep it in mind the next time you feel bound to stare at someone because they weigh much more than you do, that they are someone's son, daughter, father, mother, brother or sister – just like you are.

APPENDICES

GARY'S DIET TIPS

The most important thing to remember is that you can reach your goal weight, no matter how far off it might appear today – like me, just refuse to give up.

How you approach losing weight will be the key to your success. For instance, it should not be only about what you are losing, focus on what you will be gaining in its place. Potential transformation, emotionally and mentally, will be far greater than the sacrifice of giving up your favourite foods.

I don't believe in short-term fixes to lose weight. For me, it was about doing it properly and carefully because I wanted to change my life forever.

Diets do not work if you want to keep the weight off forever. You need to think about your entire lifestyle, and be open to making the smallest of changes that can help make the massive difference.

Changing simple bad habits can have major effects on your weight and health.

I do not believe that dieting means giving up everything you like. You will, however, have to limit what you love, for the greater good.

I cannot emphasise enough the psychological benefit of exercise.

Not only will it get you fitter and healthier, it will tone you up and, more importantly, help you feel great. Also when I was having a bad 'hunger' day, training was perfect for taking my mind of food.

Don't simply buy products just because they have the word 'Diet' on the label. Do your research and read the label carefully to make sure it really is good for you.

For me, it is not about counting calories, or subsisting on food just because it is low in calories, it is more to do with healthy eating. For example, beetroot is great for you, but I think it tastes horrible; even so I eat and drink it regularly because it makes a huge difference.

Regarding food, keep it simple. My general rule is that if my grandparents didn't eat it then I don't eat it. We eat far too much processed food and it is not good for us. Go and check out your press now and have a look at what you have bought, would your grandparents have eaten it?

You can see from the book that I believe in setting goals. After all, we all need something to motivate us, especially regarding losing weight. Whether it's to train for a marathon, or getting back into playing five-a-side with the lads, or fitting into a dress you bought a few years back, you need a reason to remember why you are doing this every single day. It might not be that important for the next person, but for you it will be a personal victory to have met it.

Trust yourself. If you feel you shouldn't be eating it, then you're probably right.

Educate yourself about the food you put into your body. This is essential to making a positive long-term change. Getting a basic understanding of protein, fats, carbohydrates, insulin levels, glycaemic index and your metabolism allows you to make better decisions.

Eat five small portions a day. Very few people know what a proper portion is; most of us simply eat more than we need to. Five small meals will prompt your metabolism to kick in much faster, helping you to lose weight.

Give it time. It will take your body about thirty days to feel the benefits from the changes in your diet, and it will also take around that amount of time before you start enjoying exercise, helping you out on the psychological front.

If you are struggling with the idea of giving up something like chocolate or wine then don't, but you could make them a 'once a week' food. You can set out your food categories:

ONCE A WEEK FOODS: Okay, this would be your wine, your burger, or whatever, along as it is incorporated in moderation, as a controlled portion to be enjoyed! Do not feel guilty for eating it; enjoy it, especially if you know you have worked hard to have it.

SOMETIME FOODS: Now, this would be stuff like fruit, which is okay to eat, just not every day because of its sugar content.

EVERYDAY FOODS: This includes vegetables, protein-rich foods, nuts and seeds.

NEVER FOODS: For me, this means the likes of a fry-up, or anything that is fried. This type of food upsets my stomach and makes me feel bad, lethargic and bloated, so it makes more sense not to eat them.

These are fairly simple tips, but they make sense to me and they have helped me get to this point. They work for me anyway and keep me from going insane!

As I finish this book, I have just finished my second Dublin marathon and taken nearly two hours off my time, we have a beautiful baby boy on the way, I am continuing my studies in college, I continue to push myself with more goals and while I have had to defer my place in the Marathon des Sables 2013 due to our baby, I will do it. I am proud to say I have realised my priorities in life, I continue to work with Chris Delooze and Nichola Forrest, I am still weighing in monthly on the *Ray D'Arcy Show* nearly twenty-two months after what I thought would be a once-off, I still have amazing support – more than I deserve – and most importantly I am very much enjoying my life.

You may be thinking, 'Why haven't you waited until your diet ends to write this book?' Well, to me the diet ended when I started working with Nichola who was the last piece in a puzzle. This is a lifestyle now.

I BELIEVE I WILL ALWAYS NEED TO WATCH MY WEIGHT CAREFULLY AND SO MY STORY HAS NO ENDING, THIS IS MERELY THE FIRST CHAPTER OF THE REST OF MY LIFE AND WE HAVE MANY EXCITING DAYS AHEAD. IF I CAN DO IT, I TRULY BELIEVE ANYBODY CAN; JUST DON'T GIVE UP ON YOURSELF AND TAKE IT DAY BY DAY. I HAVE NO REGRETS, MY PAST MAKES ME THE MAN I AM TODAY. WHILE CERTAIN PARTS OF MY LIFE EVEN NOW ARE PAINFUL TO REMEMBER, THEY MAKE ME A BETTER PERSON. I HOPE BY READING MY STORY YOU WILL SEE THAT I AM NOBODY SPECIAL, I JUST REFUSED TO GIVE UP ON MYSELF, WHICH IS FAR HARDER THAN ANYBODY CAN IMAGINE AND IS SOMETHING THAT IS ALWAYS TESTED, BUT I AM WINNING.

NUTRITIONIST NICHOLA FORREST'S TIPS

What were your first impressions of Gary?

I found him to be focused, motivated and very articulate as regards what he was looking for from me. I liked the way that he wanted to develop an understanding of how to feed himself properly using simple foods – meat, fish, vegetables, salads etc.

What do you think of Gary's training regime?

From what I know of Gary as a person, his training is fundamental to his success as it keeps him motivated to stick to strict eating habits day after day (never underestimate how hard this can be!) Everyone needs goals and some sort of a reward system and I think for Gary, the training he does supplies this. I always support exercise as part of weight loss, obviously within the parameters of a person's health and ability.

Every person who has weight to lose has challenges to meet as regards self-discipline, consistency, maintaining motivation and so on, because for the most part, they are trying to unravel lifetime habits that have led them to carrying weight in the first place. What's brilliant about Gary is that he is entirely focused, he has no interest in slipping back into old habits, he follows the rules to a tee … obviously the ideal client from my perspective!

Why did Gary need a nutritionist? What was wrong, and what could you put right?

I think the thing about nutrition and food is that everyone can have very individual needs. You know the expression 'One man's food is another man's poison'; well, I find that sometimes what looks like a perfectly sensible eating plan just isn't working for whatever reason. I try to tweak an individual's eating choices so that they feel good, they feel healthy and they are getting the results they want. This is often a case of trial and error. In Gary's case, he was eating 'healthily', but had reintroduced breads and grains into his diet and was gaining weight again. He also felt frustrated, tired and sluggish. It was only when we removed these foods and increased his consumption of salads and vegetables alongside his meat, fish, nuts, seeds, eggs etc. that he felt better and started to lose weight again.

What are your feelings about diets in general?

I don't like the word 'diet' because I think we tend to associate it with restriction, hunger, loss of enjoyment in food … The point is that nowadays we have huge amounts of food available to us, we're not programmed to say 'no' as a rule and we mostly tend to be less physically active as well. Eating well is a lifestyle and it can take time to create new habits. My main advice is to try to eat real food that came from nature as much as possible i.e. fruit, vegetables, meat, fish, nuts, seeds, wholegrains rather than processed white versions. Processed foods are unfortunately often high in salt, sugar or fat and can be less satisfying long term.

When someone is very overweight, what is the best way to go about losing weight?

Again, I don't think there is a 'one size fits all' when it comes to weight loss. I don't agree with plans that move too far away from proper food but you have to put things in context – if someone is very overweight, their health is in jeopardy and they need to change and sometimes a strict regime is the only way to start. It's important to find the reason that they gained weight and address that as well as educating them about food so as to prevent relapse!

Gary has made the point that most of us eat too much, that we know little about the proper portions? Do you agree with this, and can you say why?

I agree. Keeping a detailed food diary is often very enlightening from this perspective. My clients are often very surprised to see what they're really eating in a day. Also, exercise and proper hydration both help to regulate appetite and thus help you to eat the correct amount for your body.

As a nutritionist, is there any one thing you would like to tell people about food and food choices?

I think people can be oblivious to the fact that food choices can affect everything – how you feel, how you look, how much energy you have, how long you live … In my opinion, choosing highly-nutritious foods can improve long-term health, but so often we just eat without any thought as to whether what we're eating is good or bad and that frustrates me.

Healthy eating is also about balance. I don't particularly agree with low-fat products mainly because they have been altered from their real state and in many cases, this means something else is added like sugar in order to improve their flavour … I include olive oil, nuts, seeds, avocados as part of my recommendations for most people because they are rich in the beneficial omega fats that the body needs. Again, portions are the relevant issue here. A little of anything is generally okay. In the same way that it's not recommended to eat an entire cheesecake, but rather just a small slice as a treat, a small handful of raw nuts such as almonds or brazils is what I would be recommending, not the whole bag!

Is there a common mistake that people make, when they go on a diet?

I think their main mistake is thinking that there is a quick fix out there or that they will be able to revert to old habits without consequences ... it's all about changing for the better and sustaining that.

For someone wanting to lose weight, what's the most important thing to remember?

Look at the obvious things first and fix them.

Are you skipping breakfast or meals in general?

Are you eating junk?

Is there an excess of fat (chocolate, biscuits, crisps, takeaways), sugar, starchy white carbohydrates (bread, pasta, rice, potatoes) in your diet?

If not, then follow a few simple rules and see do they work:

Always eat breakfast

Eat 4–5 small meals/snacks spread out during the day

Include small amounts of protein at every meal/snack e.g. eggs, nuts, seeds, fish, meat and so on.

First published 2013 by The O'Brien Press Ltd,
12 Terenure Road East, Rathgar, Dublin 6, Ireland.
Tel: +353 1 4923333; Fax: +353 1 4922777
E-mail: books@obrien.ie
Website: www.obrien.ie
ISBN:978-1-84717-524-3
Copyright for text © Gary Kirwan 2013
Copyright for typesetting, layout, editing, design © The O'Brien Press Ltd

British Library Cataloguing-in-Publication Data
A catalogue record for this title is available from the British Library

1 2 3 4 5 6 7 8 9 10
13 14 15 16 17 18

Front cover and internal images: iStockphoto.
Back cover & internal photographs courtesy of the Kirwan Family.
Editing, typesetting, layout and design: The O'Brien Press Ltd

Printed and bound by Scandbook AB, Sweden
The paper used in this book is produced using pulp from managed forests.